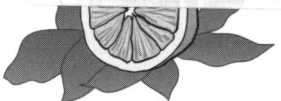

To _____

From _____

My Favorite Recipes:

Signed _____

Date _____

Library of Congress Catalog Card Number: 2009909767
ISBN: 978-0-97605-559-4

For information write to:
Famous Florida!® Enterprises, Inc.
Seaside Publishing,
P.O. Box 14441
St. Petersburg, Florida 33733
Toll Free: 888-FLA-BOOK (352-2665)

famousflorida@aol.com
www.seasidepublishing.com

Book Designer: Susannah Green
Publisher: Joyce LaFray

Printed in the United States of America

Seaside books may be purchased for business, educational or sales promotional use.

FAMOUS florida!®
Delicious
Grapefruit
Recipes

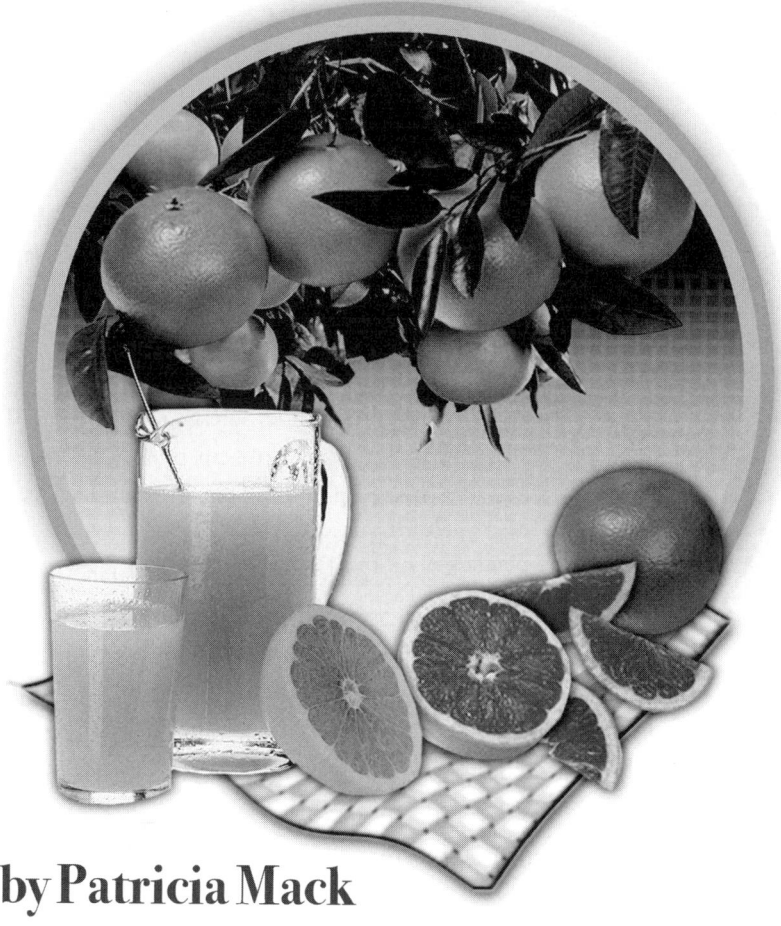

by Patricia Mack

Seaside
Publishing

This book is dedicated to my father, Henry Johnson, who taught me the wonders of living in the Sunshine State — literally and figuratively.

Patricia Mack

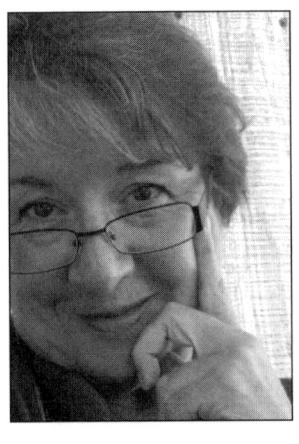

Patricia Mack, Food Writer extraordinaire, extols the outstanding taste of this scrumptious fruit, as well as the fruit's innumerable health benefits.

For instance, did you know that one-half of a medium sized fresh pink grapefruit is 60 calories? The spunky fruit also provides fiber, calcium and lycopene, a phytochemical thought to reduce chronic diseases such as cancer.

In the fourteenth of the popular Famous Florida!® series, Pat Mack takes you on a culinary tour of Florida's best grapefruit recipes. Her collection includes a variety of classics as well as popular secret recipes from some of Florida's most famous restaurants.

Table of Contents

Introduction

Coolers and Cocktails

Appetizers and Party Foods

Salads and Salad Dressings

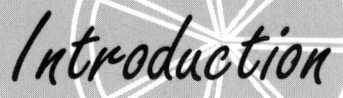

Introduction

The Citrus of Paradise

My Florida vacation home came complete: a palm tree in the front yard, a lovely lake in the back yard, and a petite grapefruit tree in the side yard. All three provide us great pleasure, but the grapefruit tree is the jewel.

As I write this, I look out my window at the yellow clusters that give the grapefruit its name, as grapefruit grow in bunches, like grapes.

Why, I wonder, does grapefruit take its name from another fruit, rather than its cousins the orange and the tangerine that have their own special moniker? Even its scientific name, *Citrus paradisi x*, sounds better than "grapefruit", translation "the citrus of paradise!"

The grapefruit is descended from the pummelo, a giant thick-skinned grapefruit from Malaysia that weighs as much as 25 pounds. The grapefruit actually developed as a hybrid of both the pummelo (Citrus maxima) and the sweet orange (*Citrus sinensis*).

Before the grapefruit became known as "grapefruit" it was called the "forbidden fruit of Barbados," named some time around the 1700s for the island where it was discovered. Thank goodness no one paid attention to the "forbidden" part! If forbidden to eat this delicious fruit, I would have missed its luscious flavor.

Transported to Florida in the late 1800s, the grapefruit found a perfect home, quickly becoming one the state's most important crops. Not surprisingly, there are a number of grapefruit varieties but you will usually find seedless or not, and white, pink or red varieties. Which is best is a matter of opinion, although the red and pink have a higher amount of vitamin A and contain the healthful anti-oxidants beta-carotene and lycopene.

In season, I pluck a fresh grapefruit from my little tree each morning to slice or squeeze for breakfast, but that doesn't put a dent into the enormous amount of fruit this prolific plant produces. Family and friends have been the recipients of teeming baskets of the fruit — on more than one occasion. I offer free access to neighbors while I enjoy my grapefruit morning, noon and night. Still, there is more left on the tree!

My cooking experiments with this luscious fruit confirm my initial hunch that grapefruit is superb in appetizers, salads, entrees, desserts and beverages. I assure you, I'm not alone in my appreciation. Sunshine State chefs, cooking professionals and home cooks have also discovered inventive, appealing and unconventional ways to incorporate this plentiful and beautiful citrus into a host of dishes. They have my gratitude for sharing their favorites on these pages.

My grapefruit tree has become synonymous with infinity and the possibilities for enjoying its marvelous fruit are truly endless.

Patricia Mack

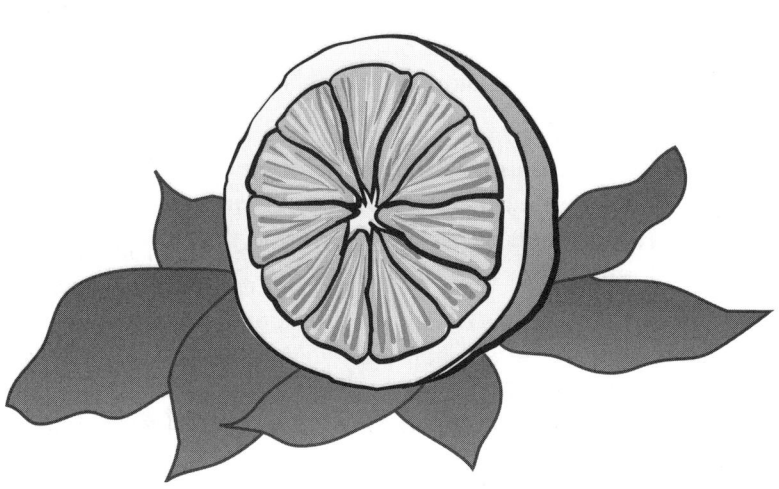

A Healthful Diet

Grapefruit provides important nutrients that help meet daily dietary requirements. A single serving contains less than 100 calories, has no fat, cholesterol or sodium. Including grapefruit in your diet will provide you with:

*Vitamin C that helps heal wounds, aids in iron absorption, and strengthens body tissues, bones and blood vessels. It is an antioxidant which helps fight the development of certain forms of cancer and heart disease.

*Folate, a B vitamin important for mature red-blood cell production and guards against anemia. It is especially important for women of childbearing age to take in plenty of folate prior to and during pregnancy.

*Potassium, an essential mineral that helps maintain fluid balance in the body, promotes cell strength, supports cell structure and nerve function.

*Fiber, abundant in the whole fruit, has been found to help prevent the development of some forms of cancer, in reducing blood-cholesterol levels and in aiding digestion and elimination.

Take Notice — There May Be Interactions For Some
Grapefruit has serious interactions with many commonly prescribed medications. This interaction can lead to unpredictable and hazardous levels of certain drugs and they should not be consumed with grapefruit unless advised by a doctor.

The Grapefruit Kitchen

Although grapefruit are available year around, the peak season for Florida grapefruit is October to June.

When choosing a grapefruit, select one that is heavy for its size, with a bright skin color, and no bruises. The grapefruit should be firm and springy when touched.

The best place to store grapefruit is in the refrigerator crisper where it will stay fresh up to a month, but please, don't put it in a plastic bag. This will result in the accumulation of too much moisture that will damage the fruit.

There are a number of grapefruit gadgets worth investing in if you have a passion for the fruit.

*A grapefruit knife is a slightly curved, serrated knife that can be slipped around a grapefruit half, and between the connective interior membranes to make eating the grapefruit easy

*A grapefruit spoon is a teaspoon with serrated edges that allows you to cut through the membrane while eating a grapefruit half.

*A zester is a small peeling instrument that can be purchased at most gourmet shops. It simplifies the task of cutting away the peel without taking any of the bitter white pith. This is the perfect instrument if you want to candy or blanche the peel for use in a recipe.

*A grater or plane grater that looks like a rasp, shreds peel into tiny bits to be thrown into batters and sautéed dishes.

The Art of Peeling

Although it is possible to peel a grapefruit as one peels an orange or a tangerine, cutting it into usable parts makes far more sense. The Florida Citrus Growers, an industry group, recommends this method:

1. With a sharp knife, slice each end off fruit.
2. Stand the fruit on one of the cut ends and slice away peel, being sure to get all the white pith.
3. Cut slices around the middle or core, which is bitter and contains seeds.
4. Then cut between membranes to free the fruit.

What is Zest?

You'll see the word "zest" in many of the recipes. Zest is the outside, colored rind of citrus fruit. It is actually the most flavorful part of the fruit and it gives food a lovely fragrance and flavor.

When removing the zest, it is important to take only the bright, shiny thin outer part of the peel. Leave the white, bitter part (the pith)

behind. You can use a zester, a fine grater, a vegetable peeler or a sharp paring knife to remove the zest.

If a recipe calls for "minced zest," stack the pieces of zest on top of one another and cut very thin slices lengthwise into strips, then chop the thin strips crosswise into very fine bits.

Grapefruit Cooking Secrets

Cooking with grapefruit all these years, I've learned a lot about how to use its wonderful flavor. Here are some basics:

- 1 medium grapefruit will yield about ⅔ cup of juice.

- Grapefruit at room temperature will yield more juice than those that are refrigerated.

- Combine equal parts of grapefruit juice with lime juice, and you replicate the taste of yuzu [YOO-zoo] a Japanese citrus fruit that is intensely sour but extremely appealing. It has become the darling of many American chefs, but is quite pricy in this country, and rarely fresh.

- Mix grapefruit with orange juice to achieve a delightful tang.

- Although lemon juice is the citrus most recommended to keep fruit from turning brown after it is cut, grapefruit juice works just as well.

- Try squeezing fresh grapefruit juice over grilled or broiled fish instead of lemon.

- Combine grapefruit sections with your favorite bagged salad, then toss with vinaigrette dressing.

- Make a "breakfast parfait" by layering strawberry yogurt, granola, and grapefruit sections.

Now, go out there and have fun with grapefruit!

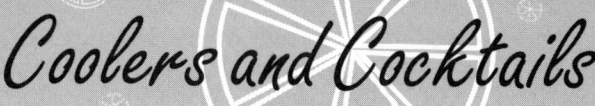

Sunshine Sangria

This is a light and refreshing version of the Spanish Sangria that we all know so well. Perfect for cooling down on a hot day, it is tantalizing poured from a clear glass pitcher into a wine goblet.

1 medium grapefruit
1 orange
2 lemons (divided use)
4 cups dry white wine such as sauvignon blanc or chablis
2 tablespoons Triple Sec (see Note)
1 tablespoon honey, preferably orange blossom
1 cinnamon stick
1 cup seedless green grapes, halved
1 quart lemon-lime carbonated soda
Ice cubes

1. Halve the grapefruit, orange and lemons.

2. Juice a grapefruit, an orange half, and a lemon. Combine and refrigerate the juice.

3. Cut the remaining grapefruit half in half again; slice the quarters into thin wedges. Cut orange and remaining lemon halves into cartwheels by slicing cross-wise.

4. Wrap citrus slices and refrigerate until ready to use.

5. Combine juices, wine, Triple Sec, honey, cinnamon stick and grapes in a large glass pitcher. Cover; refrigerate at least 1 hour.

6. Just before serving, gently stir in lemon-lime carbonated soda. Add reserved fruit slices. Add ice cubes to pitcher. Pour over ice in wine glasses.

Servings: About 12 (¾-cup each)

Note: *Triple Sec is a colorless, orange-flavored liqueur very similar to Curacao. It adds an intense citrus flavor.*

Three Classics

Grapefruit juice lends itself to many libations, but among the best-known grapefruit juice cocktails are the Greyhound, the Salty Dog and the Sea Breeze. They are served coast-to-coast, but somehow taste better in Florida bars. These recipes are from Abe & Louie's — a premier steak house in Boca Raton.

Greyhound

This grapefruit and vodka cocktail was no doubt inspired by the sleek canines that race at Florida's famous dog tracks.

1½ ounces vodka
4 ounces white grapefruit juice
Lime wedge for garnish

Yield: 1 Greyhound

1. Fill a Tom Collins glass with ice cubes.

2. Combine vodka and grapefruit juice.

3. Pour over the ice. Stir well.

4. Garnish with lime wedge.

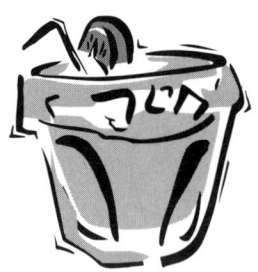

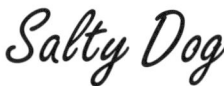

Salty Dog

This grapefruit and gin cocktail is a variation of the Greyhound but its name probably has more to do with naval history than dogs. In the navy, a "salty dog" is an experienced sailor who has traveled much and seen even more. It also carries a connotation of being a mite cantankerous.

Lime wedges (divided use)
Coarse-grained kosher salt
1½ ounces gin
4 ounces white grapefruit juice

Yield: 1 Salty Dog

1. Rub the cut edges of the lime wedge around the rim of a Tom Collins glass.
2. Pour kosher salt onto a saucer. Turn glass upside down into the salt to coat.
3. Fill glass with ice cubes.
4. Combine gin and grapefruit juice in a shaker. Shake well, and then pour over ice cubes being careful not to disturb the salt on the rim. Stir well.
5. Garnish with a lime wedge.

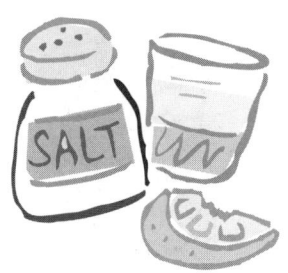

Sea Breeze

Here is a coming together of the Northern and Southern coastal states with a delicious mixture of cranberry and grapefruit juice and vodka. Use pink or Ruby Red grapefruit juice for a lovely color.

1½ ounces vodka
2 ounces cranberry juice
2 ounces grapefruit juice plus a tablespoon
Lime wedge

Yield: 1 Sea Breeze

1. Fill a Tom Collins glass with ice cubes.
2. Combine vodka and fruit juices in a shaker. Pour over the ice. Stir well.
3. Garnish with lime wedge.

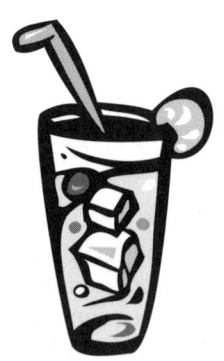

The Pink Lady

Chef Tony Acinapura became something of a hero on the reality TV show "The Restaurant" a few years ago. Acinapura, a New Yorker, relocated to Florida where he took over kitchens at Prime 707 Steakhouse & Bar in Lake Worth. Always inspired by what is freshest and best from the local market, Acinapura was impressed with the fabulous color of Florida's Ruby Red grapefruit. The result is this pretty cocktail.

Turbinado sugar (see Note 1)
**4 ounces citrus-flavored vodka such a Ketel One
  Citroen Vodka**
1 ounce Ruby Red grapefruit juice
1 tablespoon simple syrup (see Note 2)
Slender slice of Ruby Red grapefruit for garnish

1. Moisten the rim of a martini glass with a splash of grapefruit juice.

2. Sprinkle a small plate with raw sugar. Up end martini glass into the sugar to coat the rim well. Set aside.

3. Pack a cocktail shaker with ice. Add vodka, grapefruit juice and simple syrup. Shake well.

4. Pour into sugar-rimmed cocktail glass. Garnish with grapefruit slice.

Yield: 1 pink lady

Note 1: Turbinado sugar, also called "raw" sugar, is a coarse-grained sugar that is less refined than granulated sugar. It is widely available in supermarkets.

Note 2: Make simple syrup by combining 1 cup water with 1 cup granulated sugar, then heating and stirring in a saucepan over medium-high heat until sugar is completely dissolved. Cool completely at room temperature. Pour into a covered container and refrigerate. Can be stored for six months in the refrigerator.

Grapefruit Liqueur

Steeped on a kitchen countertop in an attractive wide-mouth jar with a tight fitting lid, this mixture looks so pretty you won't want to disturb it. That is until you take a sip and then you know that the only solution is to always keep a batch in process. It is delicious as an after-dinner drink or combined with lemon-lime soda and served over ice in a tall glass. Also, this is a nice gift to give during the holidays.

2 cups ginger brandy
1 grapefruit cut into 8 wedges
½ cup grapefruit juice
1 cup water
1 cup sugar

1. In a 1-quart jar, combine brandy, grapefruit wedges and grapefruit juice.

2. Cover the jar and allow the mixture to steep for 4 weeks. Occasionally shake the jar.

3. When liqueur has finished steeping, strain liquid through a strainer to remove grapefruit bits, and then set aside.

4. Combine water and sugar in 1-quart saucepan. Stir over low heat until sugar is completely dissolved. Cool.

5. Add sugar water to grapefruit brandy mixture to taste. Mix well.

6. Filter brandy and sugar water through a coffee filter into a decorative bottle with a tight seal.

Yield: About 1 quart

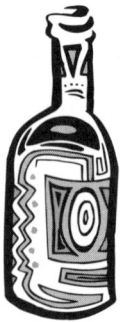

Island-Style Punch

This is a celebratory beverage. It is as stunning to see, as it is delicious to drink. Serve in a pretty cut-glass punch bowl.

Citrus Ice Ring:
1 Ruby Red grapefruit
½ dozen kumquats or whole strawberries
Small bunch lemon verbena or mint leaves

Punch:
3 cups Southern Comfort liquor
½ cup Jamaican rum
1 cup pineapple juice
1 cup Ruby Red grapefruit juice
½ cup lemon juice
2 quarts chilled champagne

1. To make the ice ring, quarter the grapefruit, and then slice quarters crosswise.
2. Place quarters in a ring mold. Dot with kumquats or whole strawberries and lemon verbena or mint leaves.
3. Pour enough water over the grapefruit, berries or kumquats and herb leaves to cover. Freeze.
4. Remove from freezer. Fill ring mold with water. Return to freezer.
5. When ready to add to the punch, remove the ice ring by running hot water over the outside of the mold.
6. To make the punch, combine Southern Comfort, rum and fruit juices.
7. Chill for at least one hour.
8. Pour into punch bowl. Add champagne. Float ice ring.

Servings: About 25

Hot Spiced Grape Grapefruit Juice

This is a lovely fall and winter beverage. Brewed with fragrant spices, this hot sipper will fill the house with a potpourri of aromas.

1½ cups white grape juice
Juice of ½ a lemon
1 cup white grapefruit juice
1 stick cinnamon
2 cloves
1 tablespoon sugar
Thin lemon slices (optional)

---

1. Combine fruit juices, cinnamon, cloves and sugar in a 1-quart saucepan.

2. Bring to a boil. Remove from heat. Strain.

3. Serve in glass teacups if you have them, or china teacups if you don't, garnished with a thin slice of lemon.

Servings: 2 to 3

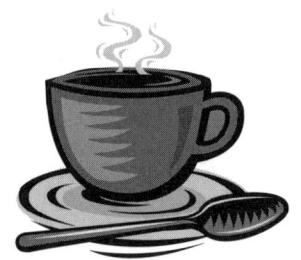

Citrus Iced Tea

Picture being barefoot on the beach as you sip this refreshing fresh-brewed ice tea on a sultry summer afternoon. The spices provide an invigorating accent, heady aroma and a deep, rich color.

1 quart boiling water
¼ cup sugar
10 whole cloves
2 cinnamon sticks, each 2-inches long
4 orange-pekoe tea bags
¼ cup white grapefruit juice
2 tablespoons lemon juice
1 tablespoon grapefruit zest
1 slice lemon
6 lemon wedges for garnish

1. Combine water, sugar, cloves and cinnamon sticks in a 2-quart saucepan.
2. Mix well and bring to a boil. Remove from heat; add tea bags. Steep 4 minutes. Strain.
3. Stir in remaining ingredients except for lemon wedges. Set aside until mixture is at room temperature.
4. Fill six tall ice tea tumblers with ice cubes. Pour tea over ice. Garnish with lemon wedges.

Servings: 6

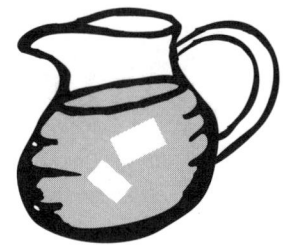

Beach Bubbly

The idea of mixing grapefruit juice and beer may seem bizarre, but the result is a rather luscious champagne-like punch. Serve it in a clear glass pitcher, adding citrus slices just before serving. They make "bubbly" look spectacular and enhance the flavor.

1 cup sugar
1 cup water
Rind of 2 lemons and 1 small grapefruit, white pith scraped
1 cup lemon juice
¾ cup grapefruit juice
1 (12-ounce) can of light beer
Lemon and grapefruit slices

1. Mix sugar with water in a saucepan.

2. Bring to a boil; add lemon and grapefruit rinds. Cover and let stand for 5 minutes.

3. Remove citrus rinds and cool to room temperature.

4. Add lemon and grapefruit juices. Pour into a large pitcher over ice.

5. Add beer and fruit slices just before serving. Stir once to mix.

Servings: 6 (½-cup each)

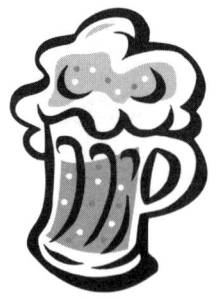

Pretty-in-Pink Grapefruit-ade

This is a drink for the ladies on a lazy high-summer afternoon. For best results, serve in clear glass tumblers. You will always remember the first taste — sweet, tart and very satisfying.

2 cups raspberries (divided use)
3½ cups water (divided use)
¾ cup extra fine sugar
1 cup pink grapefruit juice
Mint sprigs for garnish

1. Puree 1 cup of the raspberries with 1 cup of the water in a blender or food processor.

2. Force the puree through a fine sieve set over a pitcher, pressing hard on the solids.

3. Add remaining raspberries, and water, the sugar and the grapefruit juice to the pitcher.

4. Stir the mixture until the sugar is dissolved.

5. Divide among tall glasses filled with ice cubes. Garnish with mint sprigs.

Servings: 4

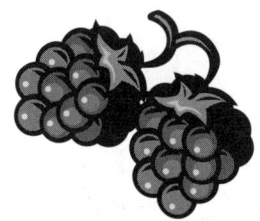

Grapefruit and Banana Smoothie

Even children will love this easy, nourishing breakfast drink. Nutritional benefits include calcium from the yogurt and milk, potassium from the bananas and vitamin C from the grapefruit juice. It's a good way to a great start in the morning. If you like your smoothies frosty, process the ingredients with a ¼ cup of crushed ice

1 (14-ounce) can sweetened condensed milk
1 (8-ounce) container banana yogurt
2 ripe bananas
½ cup grapefruit juice

1. Process all ingredients in blender or food processor until smooth, stopping to scrape down the sides.

2. Serve immediately.

Servings: 4

Chalet Suzanne's Broiled Grapefruit & Chicken Livers

For more than 70 years this dish has been the featured appetizer at Chalet Suzanne's six-course Candlelight Dinner. It was created accidentally when the legendary Clementine Paddleford, food editor at the New York Herald Tribune, dined at the Lake Wales, Florida restaurant and inn. Grilled chicken livers were on the menu as an hors d'oeuvre but they weren't ready on time. So, when the first course, broiled grapefruit, was to be served, Chalet owner, Vita Hinshaw, garnished each grapefruit with a grilled chicken liver.

2 grapefruit, at room temperature
3 tablespoons butter
1 teaspoons sugar
4 tablespoons cinnamon-sugar mixture (combine
   1 tablespoon of cinnamon with 3 tablespoons of sugar)
4 grilled chicken livers (see Note)

1. Slice grapefruit in half and cut away membrane around center of fruit.
2. Cut around each section half, close to membrane, so that the fruit is completely loosened from its shell.
3. Fill the center of each half with 1½ tablespoons butter. Sprinkle each half with a ½ teaspoon sugar, then 1 tablespoon cinnamon-sugar mixture.
4. Place grapefruit on shallow baking pan and broil just long enough to brown tops and heat to bubbling hot. Remove from oven.
5. Place a grilled chicken liver on the center of each grapefruit.

Servings: 4

Note: *To grill the chicken livers, halve each liver, trim excess membrane, and pat dry. Spray grill with non-stick cooking spray or rub with a small amount of olive oil. Place the liver halves on the grill over a medium-high flame. Cook, turning occasionally, for about 5 minutes or until livers are browned and slightly stiffened.*

Grilled Fruit Shrimp Kabobs

Melon cubes and citrus segments give these appetizer kabobs beautiful color. Have guests make their own at your next backyard barbecue. It's fun and easy.

16 ripe cantaloupe 1-inch cubes
16 fresh pineapple 1-inch cubes
16 Ruby Red grapefruit segments, membranes removed
16 large deveined, shelled and cooked shrimp
¼ cup turbinado sugar or brown sugar (see Note)
¼ cup grapefruit juice
2 tablespoons fig or sherry vinegar

1. Beginning and ending with cantaloupe cubes, alternate fruits and shrimp on eight bamboo skewers that have been soaked in water for about 30 minutes.

2. Place kabobs in a glass baking dish.

3. Combine sugar, grapefruit juice and vinegar. Pour over kabobs, turning to coat well.

4. Place kabobs on barbecue grill over medium-high heat. Cook, turning often, until the glaze on the kabobs has caramelized, about 5 to 7 minutes. Watch carefully. The sugar burns quickly.

Servings: 8

Note: Turbinado sugar is less refined than white sugar and has a leasant and distinct taste. It is available in most supermarkets.

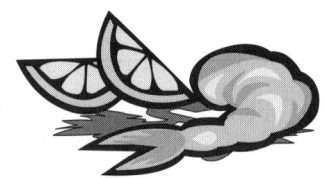

Shrimp with Grapefruit Cocktail & Louise Dipping Sauce

Louise Dipping Sauce is a take on Sauce Louise, a classic mayonnaise-based citrusy dressing that perfectly enhances the shrimp. Busy hosts and hostesses will want to know that the sauces can be made a day ahead and refrigerated, covered, until ready to serve.

1 to 1½ pounds large shrimp in shell (21 to 25 per pound count)

For Grapefruit Tomato Cocktail Sauce:
⅔ cup ketchup
⅛ teaspoon finely grated grapefruit zest
2 tablespoons grapefruit juice
1½ teaspoons fresh lemon juice
1½ tablespoons bottled horseradish sauce
¼ teaspoon hot sauce (preferably datil pepper sauce)

For Louise Dipping Sauce:
½ cup mayonnaise
2 tablespoons heavy cream
1 tablespoon grapefruit juice
½ teaspoon fresh lemon juice
½ teaspoon Worcestershire sauce
2 tablespoons scallions
2 tablespoons green bell pepper, chopped
⅛ teaspoon of hot sauce (preferably datil pepper sauce)

1. Fill a 6- to 8-quart pot two-thirds full with salted water. Bring to a boil.

2. Add shrimp and return to a simmer, stirring occasionally until shrimp are pink and almost cooked through, about 3 minutes.

3. Drain and cool. Peel shrimp, leaving tail intact.

4. Chill, covered, in the refrigerator while preparing sauces.

5. To make the grapefruit tomato cocktail sauce, stir together ketchup, grapefruit zest, fruit juices, horseradish sauce and hot sauce until well combined. Chill.

Recipe continues on next page ⊃

6. To make the Louise dipping sauce, spoon mayonnaise into a bowl. Whisk in cream and grapefruit juice, then add remaining ingredients.

7. Serve shrimp on an attractive serving platter, with bowls to hold the dipping sauces.

Servings: 4 to 6

Note: *Datil pepper sauce is a fiery condiment that historians believe was brought to St. Augustine by Minorcan settlers in the 1700s. Although it is recommended for this recipe, any hot sauce can be substituted.*

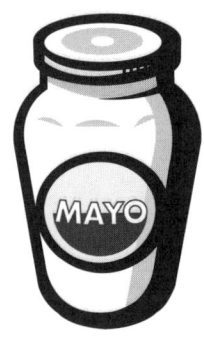

Sunshine Glazed Chicken Wings

There are many styles of chicken wings, from the basic Buffalo to Asian to Mexican. These are Florida style. They take their flavor from orange blossom honey and grapefruit. Great party fare!

2 pounds chicken wings, tips removed
⅓ cup soy sauce
⅓ cup orange blossom honey
⅓ cup grapefruit juice
1 tablespoon lemon juice
¼ teaspoon grated fresh ginger
½ teaspoon dried marjoram
1 large tomato cut into six wedges
1 medium grapefruit peeled and segments separated, membrane removed

1. Place wings in a 9" x 13" glass baking dish.

2. Combine soy, honey, fruit juices, ginger and marjoram. Pour marinade over chicken wings. Turn chicken wings to coat well.

3. Refrigerate for no less than one hour or overnight.

4. To broil, preheat broiler for 10 to 15 minutes. Remove wings from marinade and place on a broiler pan that has been prepared with non-stick cooking spray. Broil the chicken wings, four inches from the source of heat, turning once, until tender, golden brown and juices run clear, about 25 minutes.

5. While chicken wings are broiling, combine tomato and grapefruit.

6. Remove wings from the broiler. Toss with the tomato and grapefruit mixture.

7. Serve immediately.

Servings: 6

Citrus Sugared Nuts

These are positively addictive. The grapefruit juice mellows the sweetness of the sugar coating and adds a nice spike to the nuts. Set them out in little bowls so guests can nibble.

3 cups sugar
½ cup water
½ cup grapefruit juice
1 teaspoon grated grapefruit zest
1 teaspoon grated orange zest
1 pound walnuts or pecans or a combination

1. Dissolve sugar in water and grapefruit juice in a medium-size saucepan.

2. Cook to softball stage when tested in ice water, or to 238 degrees F. on a candy thermometer.

4. Remove from heat and add fruit zests and nuts.

5. Stir quickly until mixture looks chalky but is not hardened.

6. Drop by teaspoons onto oiled surface. Separate into small pieces when firm.

Yield: About 1½ pounds sugared nuts

Frozen Grapefruit Gems

These frosty confections make an unusual starter as well as a pretty, elegant and easy-to-serve party dessert. They can be made ahead and frozen. Every ingredient is a star in its own right. Yum!

1 (12-ounce) box vanilla wafer cookies
3 cups confectioners' sugar
1 (6-ounce) can frozen grapefruit juice concentrate
½ cup butter, melted
½ cup chopped pecans
½ cup flaked coconut

1. Crush vanilla wafer cookies with a rolling pin or in a food processor or blender, until finely crumbed.
2. Mix together with all ingredients except coconut.
3. Shape into small balls and roll in coconut.
4. Freeze.
5. Serve frozen in a chilled parfait glass.

Yield: About 3 dozen

Mint Grapefruit Delights

This is an unusual elegant starter. The grapefruit makes it sparkle on the palate. Everyone will ask for the recipe.

2 white grapefruit
2½ cups white grape juice
¼ pound white after-dinner mints
Fresh mint leaves

1. Pare grapefruit, removing all white pith.
2. Remove membrane from segments. Discard seeds.
3. Combine segments, juice and after-dinner mints in a large glass bowl. Cover and chill overnight.
4. Spoon into chilled sherbet glasses. Garnish with fresh mint leaves.

Servings: 6

Bananas and Sunbeam Peanut Dip

Who hasn't a favorite peanut butter combo? This one sounds like an unlikely mixture, but trust me, it is one of tastiest nibbles around.

½ **cup smooth peanut butter**
¼ **cup grapefruit juice**
2 tablespoons lime juice
2 tablespoons orange blossom honey
6 firm, ripe bananas
Chopped unsalted peanuts

1. To prepare the dip: Combine peanut butter, fruit juices and honey in a blender or food processor. Process until smooth.

2. To serve: Peel bananas. Cut into 1-inch lengths, and then slice each piece lengthwise. Arrange bananas on a serving platter with a small bowl of the dip sprinkled with chopped peanuts.

Yield: about 18 pieces

Kielbasa with Grapefruit Glaze

Kielbasa, also known as Polish sausage, is slightly less spicy but similar to andouille sausage which can also be used in this recipe. Serve in a chafing dish for maximum visual impact.

1 tablespoon canola oil
2 pounds kielbasa, sliced into 1-inch rounds
¾ **cup grapefruit or orange marmalade**
3 tablespoons (approximate) grapefruit juice

1. Warm oil in a 10-inch frying pan over medium-high heat.

2. Add kielbasa, turning with a spatula until the surfaces of the slices are crisp and browned. Carefully pour off any excess oil.

3. Add marmalade to the pan. Stir in enough grapefruit juice to melt the marmalade to a gravy consistency. Continue to simmer until mixture is smooth, turning the sausage slices frequently to prevent burning.

4. Serve with toothpicks for spearing.

Servings: 6 to 8

Grapefruit and Grouper Ceviche

Ceviche is a citrus marinated seafood salad. Most often the highly acidic marinade is made with lemons and limes, but at Chef Allen's in Aventura, Florida, award-winning chef Allen Susser adds grapefruit juice to create this distinctive dish.

- **2 pounds fresh grouper**
- **½ cup freshly squeezed lemon juice**
- **½ cup freshly squeezed lime juice**
- **1 cup freshly squeezed grapefruit juice**
- **1 medium jalapeno, seeded and minced**
- **1 large sweet red bell pepper, cut into a fine julienne**
- **1 large sweet yellow bell pepper, cut into a fine julienne**
- **1 small red onion, thinly sliced**
- **1 teaspoon minced garlic**
- **1 tablespoon kosher salt**
- **½ tablespoon freshly ground black pepper**
- **1 tablespoon fermented fish sauce (available in Asian markets)**
- **½ cup coconut milk**
- **½ cup fresh cilantro leaves**
- **1 large grapefruit, segmented and cut into pieces**

1. Cut the grouper into short, thin matchstick pieces about ⅛-inch thick.
2. Place the pieces in a stainless steel bowl.
3. Combine the lemon and lime juices. Pour over the fish, cover and refrigerate for 1 hour.
4. Drain the citrus juices, and discard. Add the grapefruit juice to the fish. Cover and refrigerate for about 15 minutes.
5. Remove bowl from the refrigerator. Add the jalapenos, peppers, onion, garlic, salt, pepper, fish sauce and the coconut milk to the grouper and grapefruit mixture.
6. Return bowl to the refrigerator, covered, for at least 30 minutes.
7. Add the cilantro and grapefruit pieces just before serving.

Servings: 4

Hint of Mint Asparagus & Grapefruit Salad

Mint is a natural with grapefruit, but a real surprise when paired with asparagus for this first course salad. The key is to toast the almonds to extract their best flavor. Remember, toasting is always done carefully — a second too long, and the almonds will burn.

½ **pound asparagus, trimmed of woody stem ends**
¼ **cup grapefruit juice**
¾ **cup chopped fresh mint, divided use**
2 **tablespoons lemon juice**
1¼ **cups vegetable oil**
¼ **cup sherry vinegar**
1 **teaspoon turbinado sugar (see Note 1)**
½ **teaspoon sea salt**
½ **cup slivered almonds, toasted (see Note 2)**

1. Cook asparagus until tender crisp in a 2-quart pot of boiling water.
2. Drain and run under cold water. Pat dry. Set aside.
3. Make the vinaigrette by combining ¼ cup grapefruit juice and ¼ cup mint in a small saucepan. Bring to a boil over medium-high heat; remove from heat. Set aside for 10 minutes then strain liquid into a mixing bowl.
4. Add to the liquid the remaining ½ cup of mint, lemon juice, oil, vinegar, sugar and salt. Whisk together until well combined.
5. Arrange the asparagus on an attractive serving platter. Drizzle with vinaigrette. Sprinkle with almonds.

Servings: 6

Note 1: Turbinado is a less refined form of sugar. It has a unique flavor, but ordinary table sugar can be used as a substitute.

Note 2: To toast almonds, place them in a dry skillet over medium heat. Roast them, watching carefully because they can easily burn, for about 4 to 5 minutes. Cool before using.

Molded Grapefruit Cabbage Salad

This is a handsome salad and one that is a cinch to tote to a large gathering or potluck dinner. It is easier to make if you purchase pre-shredded cabbage.

Salad:
1 (4-ounce) package lime gelatin
1/8 teaspoon salt
1 cup hot water
1 tablespoon lemon juice
1 large orange
1 medium grapefruit
1 cup shredded white cabbage
1 tablespoon thinly sliced scallions, white part only

Sour Cream Dressing:
1/8 teaspoon paprika
1/2 teaspoon sugar
1 teaspoon salt and dash of pepper
1 teaspoon Dijon mustard
1 cup evaporated milk
6 tablespoons grapefruit juice

1. Dissolve gelatin and salt in hot water Add lemon juice.

2. Peel and section orange and grapefruit; reserve juice.

3. Add enough water to the juice to make 1 cup, then add to gelatin mixture. Chill until slightly thickened.

4. Dice orange and grapefruit sections. Fold into gelatin along with cabbage and scallions. Turn into a 1 1/2-quart ring mold. Chill until firm.

5. To prepare the sour cream dressing, whisk together paprika, sugar, salt, pepper, mustard and milk until smooth.

6. Stir in grapefruit juice. Chill thoroughly.

7. When ready to serve, unmold the grapefruit-cabbage salad onto a serving platter that has been lined with fresh greens. Serve sour cream dressing on the side.

Servings: 7

Citrus Vinaigrette

Grapefruit provides the sassy taste note to this all-purpose salad dressing. Prepare it in a blender or food processor for best results. Be sure to use light olive oil or vegetable oil so that nothing interferes with the bright sunny flavor.

½ **cups grapefruit juice**
2 **tablespoons sherry vinegar**
2 **tablespoons balsamic vinegar**
2 **tablespoons sugar**
1 **tablespoon honey mustard**
1 **teaspoon sea salt**
½ **teaspoon freshly ground black pepper**
1½ **cup light olive oil or vegetable oil**

1. Combine all ingredients except the olive oil in a blender or food processor. With the machine running, gradually add the oil through the feedhole.

2. Process until smooth.

Yield: about 2½ cups

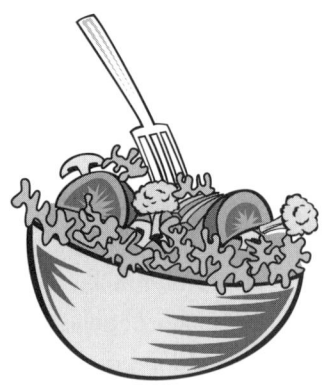

Mixed Greens & Grapefruit Avocado Dressing

Grapefruit, dried cranberries and nuts accent a creamy avocado dressing that is the crowning glory of a light and refreshing tossed salad of greens and citrus segments.

Salad:
6 cups mixed salad greens
1 medium grapefruit, peeled, sectioned and diced
¼ cup chopped pecans
2 tablespoons dried cranberries

Dressing:
1 ripe avocado, peeled, pitted and diced
1 tablespoon sherry vinegar
1 tablespoon grapefruit juice
1 teaspoon minced garlic
⅛ teaspoon ground black pepper
½ teaspoon sea salt
½ cup light olive oil

1. Place washed greens in a large salad bowl, tossing well to mix.

2. To make the dressing, combine avocado, vinegar, grapefruit juice, garlic, pepper, salt and oil in blender or food processor. Process until smooth, adding a little water if needed to reach the right creamy consistency.

3. Spoon dressing over greens, then sprinkle with grapefruit segments, pecans and cranberries.

Servings: 4

High Summer Chicken Salad

This is a main-dish salad that has unique flavor due to marinade ingredients that include ginger and grapefruit marmalade. If you can't find grapefruit marmalade, substitute orange marmalade. It will still be delicious.

Marinade:
2 tablespoons grapefruit marmalade
1 teaspoon fresh ginger, grated
1 garlic clove, chopped fine
¼ cup white wine vinegar
¼ cup grapefruit juice
¼ cup lemon juice
½ cup olive oil
Freshly ground black pepper

Chicken Salad:
4 boneless, skinless chicken breast halves (about 1 pound)
1½ cups fresh raspberries (divided use)
Assorted field greens
½ cup pecan pieces
4 (½-inch thick) grapefruit rounds, quartered

1. Combine marinade ingredients in a glass bowl or large glass jar with a tight fitting lid. Whisk or shake until ingredients are well combined.

2. Divide marinade, reserving a ½ cup for basting.

3. Grill or broil chicken 10 to 15 minutes, or until no longer pink in center and juices run clear when cut. Turn once and baste often with the reserved marinade. Cut cooked chicken into strips.

4. Discard any of the marinade used for basting.

5. To make the dressing, process 1 cup of raspberries with the remaining marinade in a food processor or blender.

6. To plate, arrange field greens on four individual serving plates. Top with chicken slices. Drizzle with the dressing. Sprinkle with pecan pieces and remaining whole berries. Garnish with quartered grapefruit rounds.

Serving: 4

Summer Day Grapefruit Salad

Could there be an easier, more flavorful or prettier salad than this one? To make it into a main dish salad, just add some chopped, cooked chicken pieces.

1 cup chopped peeled, seeded mango
1 medium grapefruit, peeled, and cut into sections (white pith removed)
1 cup seedless green grapes, halved
1 cup lemon-flavored yogurt

1. Combine mango, grapefruit and grapes in a medium salad bowl.

2. Toss gently with yogurt.

3. Serve immediately on chilled plates or refrigerate, covered until ready to serve.

Servings: 4 to 6

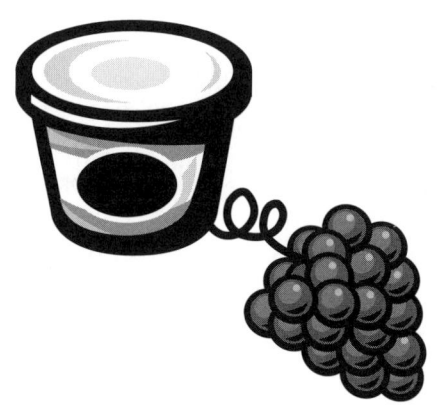

Florida Tuna Salad

This is a slightly exotic tuna salad with curry powder. Authentic Indian curry is prepared fresh daily with as many as 20 pulverized spices, but you'll find that Asian markets and even many supermarkets offer commercially prepared curry powder that is quite tasty. It comes in two styles, with Madras being the hottest.

2 (6½-ounce) cans white meat tuna
2 cups grapefruit segments
1 ripe avocado
1 tablespoons lemon juice
1 cup chopped celery
½ cup blanched slivered almonds
1½ teaspoons curry powder
½ cup whipped salad dressing such as Miracle Whip®
Salad greens such as romaine, baby spinach and frisee

1. Drain tuna.

2. Break fish into large pieces with a fork.

3. Reserve 12 grapefruit sections for garnish; cut remaining sections in half.

4. Cut avocado in half length-wise and remove seed. Peel and cut into 12 thin slices; sprinkle with lemon juice to prevent darkening.

5. Reserve 6 slices of avocado for garnish; cut remaining slices into fourths.

6. Combine grapefruit, avocado, celery, almonds and tuna in a medium bowl.

7. In another bowl, combine curry powder and whipped salad dressing. Pour over tuna mixture and blend lightly. Chill.

8. Serve on salad greens garnished with grapefruit and avocado slices.

Servings: 6

Red and Green Salad

The combination of red onion and grapefruit may at first appear to be an odd pairing, but sliced grapefruit and paper-thin rings of mild red onion work deliciously.

6 cups Italian blend salad greens
2 Ruby Red grapefruit
½ cup paper-thin slices of red onion rings
3 tablespoon Ruby Red grapefruit juice
¼ cup extra virgin olive oil
1 teaspoon seasoned salt
½ teaspoon dry mustard
1 teaspoon sugar

1. Place greens in a salad bowl.

2. Peel grapefruit, taking care to remove all the white pith. Cut in half lengthwise, and then slice into thin crosswise slices.

3. Arrange over salad greens; top with onion rings.

4. Combine remaining ingredients in a blender, food processor or jar with a tight fitting lid. Process or shake until well mixed.

5. Spoon over salad ingredients just before serving.

Servings: 8

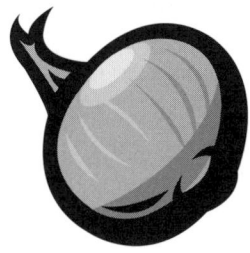

Grapefruit, Fennel & Watercress Salad

This is a composed salad – which means the ingredients are artfully arranged rather than tossed in a jumble. There are few ingredients but each one has a unique taste and color: the deep green watercress is pungent with a slight peppery snap; pale yellow grapefruit is astringent and tangy and the delicate, lime-tinted fennel brings warmth and a slight sweetness.

2 heads fennel, feathery fronds removed
1 medium seedless grapefruit
2 bunches watercress
2 lemons
¼ cup extra virgin olive oil
Salt and pepper

1. Halve, core, and thinly slice fennel. Set aside.

2. Peel and segment grapefruit. Set aside.

3. Clean and pick over watercress.

4. Zest lemon rind and juice the lemons. Whisk together lemon juice, zest and olive oil. Season to taste. Add any excess juice from grapefruit to the dressing.

5. Toss small amount of the dressing with fennel.

6. Divide fennel among four individual salad plates.

7. Toss watercress in remaining dressing and season to taste. Add to the plates.

8. Arrange grapefruit segments on top of greens.

Servings: 4

Spiny Lobster Chunks with Grapefruit Cocktail

Home economists at the Florida Department of Agriculture and Consumer Services devised this appealing salad made with peppery baby arugula and buttery avocado. Visit the department's Web site, www.FL-Seafood.com, for excellent seafood recipes like this one.

4 teaspoons shallots, finely chopped
4 tablespoons fresh lemon juice
½ teaspoon salt
6 tablespoons extra-virgin olive oil
3 cups spiny lobster meat, cooked and chilled (see Note)
4 cups baby arugula
2 ripe avocadoes, halved, peeled and sliced
2 small pink grapefruit, peeled and sectioned
Sea salt to taste

1. Combine shallots, lemon juice, and salt in a small bowl. Add oil in a steady stream, whisking to blend. Set aside.

2. Slice cooked lobster meat into ½-inch-thick medallions.

3. Arrange arugula, avocado slices, lobster slices and grapefruit sections on 4 salad plates; drizzle with shallot-lemon dressing. Add sea salt to taste.

Servings: 4

Note: *The spiny lobster, also known as the rock lobster, is Florida and the Caribbean's native lobster. It lacks the massive claws of its New England cousin. The tail meat is firmer and not as sweet.*

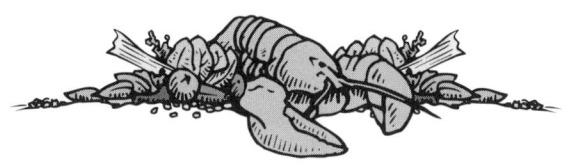

Zesty Citrus Grouper

According to Florida's Bureau of Seafood and Aquaculture Marketing in Tallahassee, the general rule for cooking fish is 10 minutes per inch of thickness at the thickest part of the fillet or fish steak at 400 to 450 degrees F. So you can see that preparing this dish, redolent with citrusy flavors, is very quick indeed.

6 Florida grouper fillets (4½ to 5 ounces each)
2 tablespoons canola oil
½ cup finely chopped onion
2 cloves garlic, minced
2 tablespoons flat-leaf parsley
1 teaspoon sea salt
⅛ teaspoon fresh ground black pepper
½ cup grapefruit juice
1 tablespoon lemon juice
1 hard cooked egg, peeled and cut into 6 wedges
6 thinly sliced grapefruit wedges with peel

1. Preheat oven to 400 degrees F.

2. Cut fish in serving sized portions and arrange in a buttered 13" x 9" x 2" glass baking dish that has been sprayed with non-stick cooking spray. Set aside.

3. Heat oil in a 10-inch skillet over medium-high heat. Add onion and garlic, cooking until transparent, about 2 minutes. Stir in parsley and salt and pepper.

4. Remove from skillet and spread mixture over fish with a spatula.

5. Combine grapefruit and lemon juice. Pour evenly over all.

6. Bake fish covered for 15 to 25 minutes, depending on thickness of the grouper, or until fish flakes easily when tested with a fork.

7. Arrange egg wedges over fish and sprinkle with paprika. Garnish with grapefruit wedges.

Servings: 6

Fabulous Florida Flounder

Two Florida ingredients – grapefruit and flounder – are combined in this savory fish dish. Thyme – called for in a very small amount – provides a big, refreshing minty nose.

6 flounder fillets (4½ to 5 ounces each)
1 teaspoon salt
⅛ teaspoon ground black pepper
¾ cup soft breadcrumbs
3 tablespoons butter, melted (divided use)
¼ teaspoon thyme leaves
12 fresh grapefruit segments, skin, pith and membrane removed

1. Preheat oven to 350 degrees F.

2. Sprinkle fillets with salt and pepper. Place in a buttered 13" × 9" × 2" glass baking dish.

3. Combine breadcrumbs with 2 tablespoons of melted butter and thyme leaves. Drizzle over fish. Top with grapefruit segments. Brush with remaining butter.

4. Bake for 35 minutes or until fish is flaky.

5. Place under broiler to brown, 3 to 4 minutes. Watch carefully so the fish does not burn.

Servings: 6

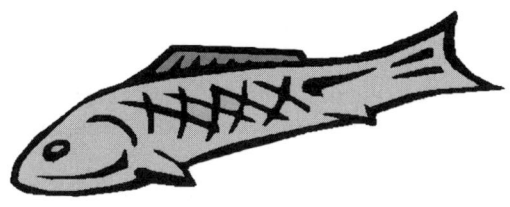

Grilled Red Snapper with Tartar Sauce

Marinades perform two important tasks: They tenderize and add extra flavor. Follow my directions correctly, and the fish will virtually melt in your mouth.

6 red snapper fillets (4½ to 5 ounces each)

Marinade:
¾ cup grapefruit juice
1 teaspoon grapefruit zest
¼ cup vegetable oil
¼ cup dry vermouth
½ teaspoon salt
Fresh ground black pepper, to taste
2 cloves garlic, minced

Grapefruit Sauce:
1 cup mayonnaise
1 tablespoon bottled capers, chopped
¼ cup grapefruit juice
1 teaspoon Dijon mustard
1 teaspoon salt
⅛ teaspoon pepper
Grapefruit segments for garnish

1. Place fillets in a buttered 13" x 9" x 2" glass dish.

2. Combine grapefruit juice, zest, oil, vermouth, salt, pepper and garlic. Pour over snapper fillets then marinate 30 minutes at room temperature.

3. Meanwhile, make sauce. Combine mayonnaise, capers, juice, mustard, salt and pepper; mix well. Refrigerate until ready to use.

Recipe continues on next page ⊃

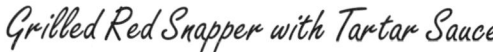

4. To cook fillets, remove fish from marinade and place in a well greased hinged, wire grill basket or on a sheet of heavy-duty aluminum foil that has been placed on top of the grill. Grill fish 3 to 4 inches above hot coals for 12 to 15 minutes, until fish flakes.

5. Remove fish to a serving platter and garnish with grapefruit wedges. Serve grapefruit sauce on the side.

Servings: 4 to 6

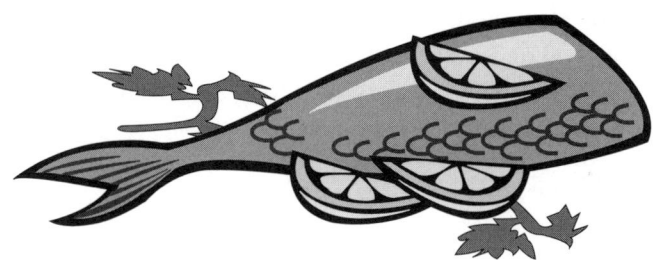

Trout with Rice Stuffing

Florida is a peninsula with vast coastlines east, south and west, so access to fresh ocean seafood is dazzling. Even Florida's interior yields some fine, sweet fresh water fish such as trout. Try this recipe that is almost a meal in itself. If you can find pecan rice, a variety sold in many supermarkets (it has no pecans but a subtle natural pecan flavor), use it!

Trout:
6 (8 to 10 ounces each) pan-dressed trout
2 teaspoons salt
Grapefruit rice stuffing (recipe follows)

Citrus Oil:
2 tablespoons canola oil
1 tablespoon grapefruit juice
1 tablespoon lemon juice

1. Preheat oven to 350 degrees F.

2. Sprinkle trout inside and out with salt.

3. Stuff fish with grapefruit rice. Close with skewers or toothpicks then place fish on a well-greased 14" x 11" x 1" baking pan.

4. Combine oil and fruit juices. Brush fish with mixture.

5. Bake for 25 to 35 minutes or until fish flakes easily when tested with a fork. Baste occasionally with citrus oil

Servings: 6

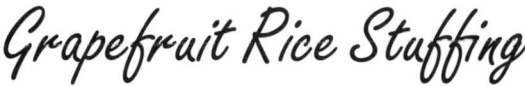

Grapefruit Rice Stuffing

Seafood stuffed with this savory mixture gives an extra dimension to the dish. It can also be served on its own as a side dish.

¼ cup butter
1 cup minced celery
1 cup minced carrot
¼ cup thinly sliced scallions, white part only
¾ cup water
¼ cup grapefruit juice
2 tablespoons lemon juice
1 tablespoon grapefruit zest
¾ teaspoon salt
1 cup instant rice
⅛ teaspoon fresh ground black pepper
¼ teaspoon thyme
½ cup chopped grapefruit segments

1. Melt butter in a 10-inch frying pan over medium-high heat.

2. Add celery, carrots and scallions. Sauté until tender, about 5 minutes.

3. Add water, juices, zest and salt; bring to a boil.

4. Add rice; stir to moisten. Cover and remove from heat. Let stand 5 minutes.

5. Stir in black pepper, thyme and grapefruit.

Yield: About 3 cups

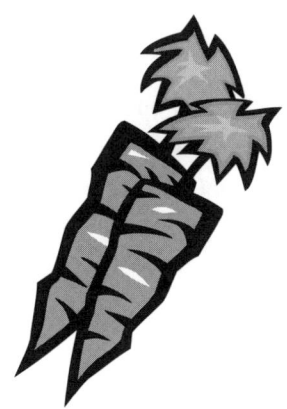

Blue Crab Cakes with Citrus Beurre Blanc

There are as many recipes for crab cakes as there are chefs, but we especially like this recipe from Tim Creehan, owner of Tim Creehan's Beach Walk at the Inn at Crystal Beach in Destin, Fla. It's simple and straight forward, and the perfect foil for the chef's buttery smooth and supple citrus beurre blanc.

2½ cups citrus beurre blanc, divided use (recipe follows)
½ medium onion, finely chopped
1 tablespoon chopped garlic
1 tablespoon chopped parsley
1 teaspoon salt
1 teaspoon freshly ground black pepper
1½ pounds jumbo lump crabmeat, picked over for shell
2 cups plain breadcrumbs (divided use)
¼ cup melted butter (for brushing onto baking sheet)

1. Preheat oven to 350 degrees F.

2. In a large mixing bowl, combine ¾ cup of the beurre blanc, onion, garlic, parsley, salt and pepper. Mix well.

3. Add the crabmeat taking care not to break it up too much. (The texture will be better if the crab is chunky.)

4. Fold in 1 cup of the breadcrumbs.

5. Spoon mixture into a 3-ounce ladle and level the top. Roll each portion in the remaining 1 cup of breadcrumbs. Form into a patty.

6. Place onto a baking sheet that has been brushed with butter. Bake for 10 minutes, turning once.

7. Serve immediately dressed with remaining citrus beurre blanc.

Servings: 4

Citrus Beurre Blanc

"Beurre blanc," pronounced *"bur-blahngk,"* is a classic French reduction sauce made with wine vinegar and shallots. These are cooked with butter and beaten until thick and foamy. The result is airy and luscious.

1 cup dry white wine such as sauvignon blanc or chablis
1 cup orange juice
1 cup grapefruit juice
1 teaspoon chopped garlic
½ teaspoon peppercorns
½ cup heavy cream
Salt and pepper, to taste
1½ pounds unsalted butter, cut into tablespoon-size pieces and chilled

1. Boil wine, fruit juices, garlic and peppercorns in a 2- to 3-quart heavy saucepan over moderate heat until liquid is syrupy and reduced 75 percent.

2. Add the heavy cream and continue to cook and stir until reduced 50 percent.

3. Add salt to taste.

4. Reduce heat to moderately low and add a few tablespoons butter, whisking constantly. Add remaining butter a few pieces at a time, whisking constantly and adding new pieces before previous ones have completely melted and the sauce is smooth and creamy.

5. Lift pan from heat occasionally to cool mixture.

6. Remove from heat; season to taste with salt and pepper.

7. Pour sauce through a medium-mesh sieve into a sauceboat, pressing on and then discarding garlic and peppercorns.

Yield: About 2½ cups

Spiny Lobster with Grapefruit Butter

The Florida Department of Agriculture and Consumer Services offers this advice on eating Florida's native lobster: Twist the head and pull to break apart from the tail. Cut the shell along the back of the tail then break from the head to the tip of the tail. Gently remove meat from the shell. Remove the sand vein by making a shallow cut along the back of the tail and rinsing under cold running water.

4 spiny lobsters, 1 ¼ to 1 ½ pounds, fresh or thawed
3 tablespoons salt
Grapefruit butter (recipe follows)

1. Bring 12 quarts of water with salt to a boil in a large saucepan or stockpot with a tight fitting lid.

2. Place lobsters in boiling water; cover and return to boiling point. Reduce heat; simmer 12 to 15 minutes. Larger lobsters will take a little more cooking time.

3. Drain; rinse with cold water for 1 to 2 minutes.

4. Split and clean lobsters. Serve with grapefruit butter.

Servings: 4

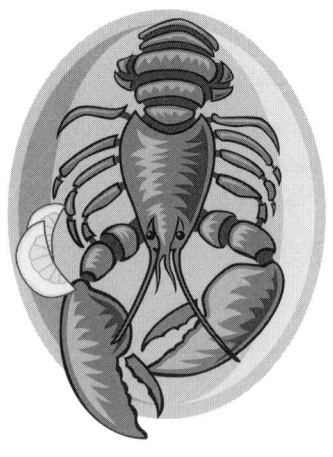

Grapefruit Butter

Grapefruit butter has only 5 ingredients, yet it produces a dynamic addition to grilled steak, seafood, pork or chicken. It takes only minutes to make, and once tasted, you'll find it's indispensable.

1 cup melted butter
2 tablespoon grapefruit juice
2 cloves garlic, pressed
2 tablespoon grated onion
Dash of datil pepper sauce or favorite hot pepper sauce (see Note)

1. Combine butter, juices, garlic, grated onion and hot sauce.

2. Mix well.

Yield: About 1 cup

Note: Datil pepper sauce is a fiery condiment that historians believe was brought to St. Augustine by Minorcan settlers in the 1700s.

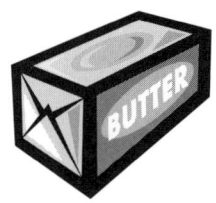

Pecan Shrimp with Dipping Sauce

Florida's wild shrimp catch is famous for its succulent, tender qualities. Residents and visitors flock to places such as Dixie Crossroads in Titusville to consume mountains of shrimp brought in by local fishermen. This recipe is an easy preparation that offers a symphony of tastes and textures with every bite.

Pecan Shrimp:
2 pounds large shrimp
¼ cup salad oil (divided use)
1 cup pecan pieces

Marmalade Dipping Sauce:
⅛ cup grapefruit or orange marmalade
¼ cup grapefruit juice
1 tablespoon lemon juice
¼ cup soy sauce
1 clove garlic, finely chopped
1 teaspoon grated fresh ginger
1 teaspoon cornstarch
1 tablespoon cold water

1. Preheat oven to 450 degrees F.

2. Butterfly shrimp by cutting lengthwise from top to tail, almost all the way through. The shrimp should lay flat, without separating.

3. Coat the shrimp with half the salad oil. Set aside.

4. Chop the pecans to a very fine powder in a food processor or blender, being careful not to over process or the pecans will become pecan butter. Spread chopped nuts in a large baking dish or on a cookie sheet.

5. Dredge the shrimp through the ground nuts. Be sure to coat each shrimp completely. Refrigerate for 5 minutes.

6. Coat a baking sheet with the remaining oil and preheat it in the oven for 2 to 3 minutes. Remove the pan from the oven and place the shrimp on it; return to the oven.

7. Roast shrimp for 5 to 7 minutes, turning once, until they are browned and firm to the touch.

Recipe continues on next page ⊃

8. While the shrimp are in the oven, combine marmalade, fruit juices, soy, garlic and ginger in a 1-quart saucepan. Bring to the boiling point. Dissolve cornstarch in cold water. Add to hot sauce and cook until thickened, two to three minutes, stirring constantly. Serve hot with pecan shrimp.

Servings: 4

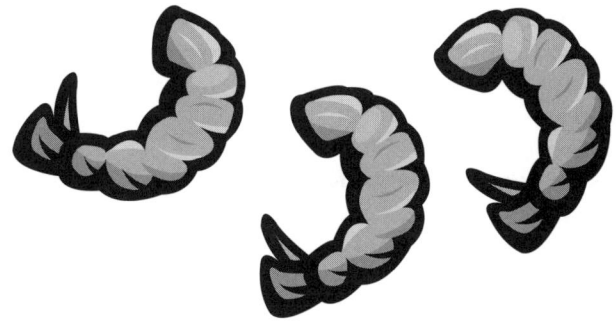

Browned Oysters on Sourdough Toast

Oysters feed mainly on single-cell plants and flourish in Florida's estuaries where nutrient-rich fresh water rivers meet coastal saltwater. Along Florida's Gulf Coast, bay men harvest oysters in small boats, using large, long-handled tongs to scoop them from the sandy bottom beds.

1 quart shucked oysters
Flour for dredging plus 1½ tablespoons for sauce
2 tablespoons butter plus a little more as needed
3 tablespoons grapefruit juice
1 teaspoon lemon juice
Worcestershire sauce
4 slices sourdough bread, toasted and then cut into toast points
Salt and pepper to taste
Parsley
Grapefruit segments

1. Drain oysters, dredge in flour and brown in 2 tablespoons butter that have been melted over medium-high heat. Remove oysters from pan with a slotted spoon; keep warm.

2. Brown 1½ tablespoons flour in pan juices, adding a bit more butter if needed.

3. Stir in any liquid accumulated around cooked oysters, grapefruit and lemon juices and a few drops of Worcestershire sauce.

4. Season with salt and pepper. Heat to boiling. Stir well until sauce is smooth; remove from source of heat.

5. Arrange toast points on individual serving dishes. Place oysters on toast and pour sauce over them. Garnish with parsley and grapefruit segments.

Servings: 4

Rock Shrimp with Cucumber Sauce

Rock shrimp are luscious little nuggets. They cook quickly, so keep a careful eye on the stove when you are preparing this dish. The cucumber sauce provides a cooling note to this delicious entree.

Cucumber Sauce:
1 cup peeled and chopped cucumber
2 tablespoons butter
2 tablespoons flour
1 cup fish stock
2 teaspoons grapefruit juice
1 teaspoon grapefruit zest
½ teaspoon grated onion
½ teaspoon sea salt

Rock Shrimp:
2 tablespoons butter
4 scallions, sliced thin, white part only
1 pound rock shrimp
¼ cup grapefruit juice
2 teaspoons lemon juice

1. To make the cucumber sauce, place cucumber with enough water to cover in a 1-quart saucepan.

2. Cook over medium-high heat until tender, about 5 minutes. Drain; set aside.

3. Wipe out the saucepan, return to source of heat, add butter and melt over medium heat.

4. Sprinkle in flour and a little of the fish stock; whisk to combine. Add more fish stock, whisking after each addition. When thick, add grapefruit juice, zest, onion and salt. Add cooked cucumber last. Remove from heat; set aside.

5. To cook rock shrimp, melt butter in a 10-inch skillet over medium-high heat. Add scallions. Sauté for 1 minute. Add rock shrimp. Sauté for 1 minute more. Add fruit juices. Bring to a boil, reduce heat and simmer 1 more minute, or until slightly thick.

6. Remove shrimp from the pan. Turn off heat.

Recipe continues on next page ⊃

7. Combine cucumber sauce with pan juices stirring well to incorporate.

8. Arrange shrimp on an attractive serving dish. Spoon sauce into a small bowl, which can also be placed on the serving dish next to the shrimp for easy dipping.

Servings: 4

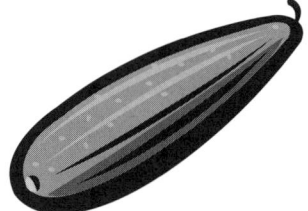

Poultry

Cornish Game Hens with Sweet and Sassy Sauce

The combined flavors of honey, ginger and grapefruit are ambrosia, but wait until you see the magnificent color of these roasted game hens when they come out of the oven. This is the dish that will make guests "ohh" and "ahh." Game hens, sold in most supermarket poultry sections, are really miniature chickens – hybrids of Cornish and White Rock chicken.

Stuffing:
1 tablespoon butter
½ cup minced celery
½ cup blanched almonds, chopped
1 cup wild rice, cooked

Game Hens:
4 game hens
Sea salt

Sweet and Sassy Sauce:
6 tablespoons thinly slivered grapefruit zest
¾ cup grapefruit juice
1½ cups honey, preferably orange blossom
¾ teaspoon chopped fresh ginger

1. Preheat oven to 325 degrees F.

2. Melt butter in a 10-inch skillet over medium heat. Add celery; sauté for about 5 minutes until soft. Add almonds; heat through about 2 minutes.

3. Toss with wild rice.

4. Lightly stuff each hen with the rice mixture. Salt the hens sparsely, but do not put oil or butter on the skin, as the Sweet and Sassy Sauce will not adhere.

Recipe continues on next page ⊃

5. Spray a 9" × 13" × 2" baking pan with non-stick cooking spray. Place the chickens in the roasting pan. Roast covered for an hour.

6. While hens are roasting, combine sauce ingredients in a 1-quart saucepan over medium heat, stirring until well combined.

7. Reserve ¾ cup of the sauce.

8. Uncover hens and use remaining sauce to baste. Continue roasting, uncovered for another 30 minutes, basting every 10 minutes with the sauce. Take care when basting because the honey can burn very quickly.

9. Serve hens with the reserved sauce on the side.

Servings: 4 for hearty eaters; 8 for medium eaters

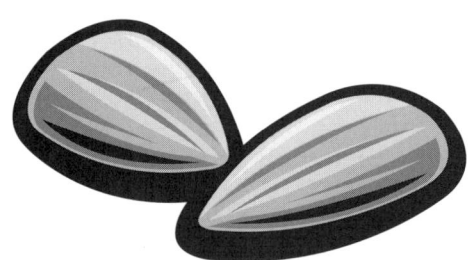

Chicken Floridian

This is a light, herbal chicken dish that is enhanced by the beautiful citrus notes derived from fresh grapefruit. Each of the herbs adds a distinctive but harmonious flavor: parsley brings a touch of pepper; rosemary adds a hint of lemony pine; and tarragon gives a soft anise taste.

2 tablespoons butter
1 tablespoon vegetable oil
6 chicken breasts quarters, dredged in flour
¼ cup chopped scallion, white and soft green parts
1 cup Rhine wine or other slightly sweet vintage
⅓ cup white grapefruit juice
1 tablespoon grapefruit zest
1 teaspoon flat-leaf parsley
2 teaspoons fresh rosemary
2 teaspoons tarragon
1 cup light cream
1 teaspoon seasoned salt
White grapefruit segments

1. Combine butter and vegetable oil in a 10-inch skillet over medium-high heat.

2. Add chicken and sauté until skin is golden. Add scallions and sauté for 1 minute more. Add wine, grapefruit juice, zest and herbs. Cover, lower heat and simmer for 40 minutes.

3. Remove chicken from pan. Keep warm on a serving plate.

4. Add cream and seasoned salt to the pan drippings, stirring to loosen brown bits. Increase heat to medium high, stirring constantly until slightly thickened.

5. Ladle some over chicken; serve remaining sauce in a gravy boat. Garnish the platter with grapefruit segments.

Servings: 6

Matchstick Chicken

Frugal cooks will appreciate using a whole chicken in this recipe. The cooking time is long, but not prep, thanks to the food processor's shredding or julienne disk. It makes quick work of chopping the vegetables so necessary as aromatics in this dish.

1 (2½- to 3-pound) roasting chicken
Coarse sea salt
Butter
½ cup julienne carrots
½ cup julienne celery
½ cup julienne onions
½ cup sliced mushroom
3 tablespoons butter
3 tablespoons flour
2½ cups chicken stock
½ cup dry white wine or dry vermouth
½ cup grapefruit juice
Peel from half a grapefruit, sliced into ribbons, pith scraped off

1. Preheat oven to 425 degrees F.

2. Rub chicken generously with salt and butter.

3. Place chicken on a rack in a roasting pan, and bake for 10 to 12 minutes, until golden.

4. Meanwhile, melt 3 tablespoons butter over medium heat in a 10" frying pan. Add vegetables when butter bubbles; sauté until vegetables soften, about five minutes.

5. Whisk in flour then add chicken stock, vermouth, grapefruit juice and peel. Simmer for 2 minutes more.

6. Pour over the chicken, cover. Lower heat in oven to 350 degrees F. and continue to roast for 40 to 50 minutes or until chicken is done.

7. Remove from oven and allow chicken to rest for about 10 minutes.

Recipe continues on next page ↪

8. Drain off pan drippings, scraping bottom to loosen the brown bits; strain through a medium sieve. Allow roasted chicken to rest for several minutes.

9. Pour off the fat that separates from the pan juices.

10. Serve carved chicken with pan juices.

Servings: 6

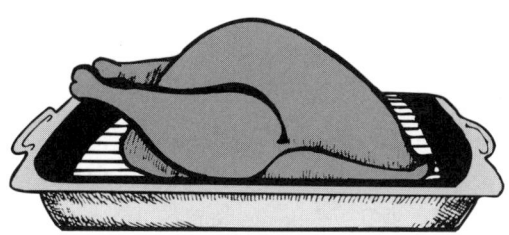

Chicken Sunny Side

These unusual ingredients bring compliments and comments. Every-one will want to know what gives this dish such a light and lively taste — the answer: grapefruit, of course. Chicken sunny side is best served with simple accompaniments such as rice and tossed salad.

- 1 broiler/fryer cut into serving pieces
- 1 cup flour mixed with salt, pepper and paprika
- ¼ cup sunflower oil
- 1 small onion, peeled and chopped
- ¼ teaspoon ground ginger
- 1 (4-ounce) can frozen grapefruit juice concentrate, thawed
- ½ cup ginger ale

1. Preheat oven to 375 degrees F.
2. Dredge chicken through seasoned flour, coating evenly.
3. Heat oil in a 10" skillet over medium-high heat.
4. Add chicken, and fry, turning frequently until golden brown.
5. Lower heat; add onion. Sauté for about 2 minutes more. Dust with ginger, turn, dust again, and turn.
6. Remove chicken and onion from pan. Place in a baking dish.
7. Combine grapefruit juice concentrate and ginger ale. Pour over chicken. Bake in a covered pan for 1 hour.
8. Remove cover. Spoon sauce from pan over chicken and continue to roast, uncovered for another 10 minutes.

Servings: 4

Grilled Chicken Thighs with Grapefruit, Garlic and Marjoram

Grilled grapefruit is a novelty, but it won't be for long once you taste how delicious — it is warm and juicy from the fire.

1 whole grapefruit

Chicken:
1½ tablespoons olive oil
2 tablespoons grapefruit juice
½ teaspoon marjoram
8 boneless, skinless chicken thighs
Salt and pepper

Sauce:
¼ cup grapefruit juice
¼ cup marjoram
1 tablespoon lime juice
2 tablespoons minced garlic
2 tablespoons coarse sea salt
2 teaspoons black pepper
⅓ cup olive oil

1. Place grapefruit in a 1-quart saucepan. Cover with water and bring to a boil.

2. Lower heat and simmer for about 20 minutes, adding more water if needed. Drain and set aside.

3. Meanwhile, in a shallow dish, whisk together olive oil, grapefruit juice, and marjoram.

4. Add chicken; turn to coat evenly. Sprinkle with salt and pepper. Cover and refrigerate for 30 minutes.

5. Meanwhile, whisk together sauce ingredients except for the olive oil. When well blended, add olive oil in a slow, steady stream as you continue to whisk. Set aside.

6. Preheat a gas grill or prepare a charcoal grill. Cut grapefruit in half, then cut the halves into quarters. Set the pieces on a grill, about 5 inches from source of heat, for about 10 minutes. Turn often so all sides hit the grid.

Recipe continues on next page ⊃

7. Remove chicken from the marinade. Place on the grill next to the grapefruit. Cook six to eight minutes on each side until juices run clear and chicken is no longer pink inside, and exterior is nicely browned.

8. Turn grapefruit and brush with the grapefruit sauce.

9. Remove chicken from the grill. Transfer to the bowl with the grapefruit sauce, turn each piece to coat, and then place on serving platter.

10. Remove grapefruit quarters from the grill and add to the serving platter. Serve with additional sauce.

Servings: 4

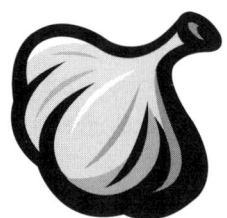

Slow-cooked Asian Chicken with Grapefruit Sauce

Frozen stir-fry vegetables make easy work of this quick and colorful dish. Serve it over vermicelli or rice noodles, for a meal.

1 (16-ounce) package frozen stir-fry vegetable mix
(broccoli, baby carrots, pea pods, water chestnuts)
1 pound skinless, boneless chicken breast halves cut into
1-inch pieces
¾ cup chicken broth
3 tablespoons grapefruit marmalade
2 tablespoons bottled teriyaki sauce
1 tablespoon grapefruit juice
1 teaspoon dry Chinese mustard
1 teaspoon 5-spice powder
1 teaspoon cornstarch
1 tablespoon water

1. Place frozen vegetables in a 3½- or 4-quart slow cooker. Place chicken pieces on top of vegetables.

2. In a small bowl combine broth, marmalade, teriyaki sauce, grapefruit juice, mustard and 5-spice powder. Pour over chicken and vegetables. Cover; cook on low for 4 to 5 hours or on high heat 2 to 2½ hours.

3. Remove meat and vegetables to a serving platter.

4. Combine cornstarch and water until well mixed. Stir into pot juices. If slow cooker is on low setting, reset it to high. Stir frequently for a few minutes until pot juices are slightly thickened. Ladle over meat and vegetables.

Servings: 4

Turkey Breast Basted in Sunlight

The Asian chili, redolent with garlic, brings a touch of oriental style and unique robust flavor to this unusual citrusy sauce.

Sunlight Sauce:
½ teaspoon grapefruit zest
⅓ cup grapefruit juice
½ cup rice wine or dry sherry
1 tablespoon oyster sauce
½ teaspoon sugar
¼ teaspoon Asian chili sauce

Turkey Breast:
1 (4- to 5-pound) fresh or frozen whole turkey breast, thawed, skin removed
Salt and pepper to taste

1. In a small bowl combine the sauce ingredients; refrigerate.
2. Heat gas or charcoal grill for indirect cooking as instructed by manufacturer. When grill is heated, carefully oil grill rack.
3. Place turkey breast on grill directly over a drip pan. Insert meat thermometer into thickest part of breast.
4. Brush turkey with Sunlight Sauce and continue to baste occasionally throughout cooking time. Cover grill; cook 1 to 1½ hours or until thermometer registers 170 degrees F. and juices run clear when pierced with fork.
5. Remove turkey breast from the grill. Let stand 15 minutes before slicing. Season to taste with salt and pepper.

Servings: 10

Fragrant Chicken Kabobs with Grapefruit Dipping Sauce

Grapefruit and ginger combine to add a warm and spicy taste to these easy-to-assemble kabobs.

Marinade:
2 tablespoons soy sauce
2 tablespoons grapefruit juice
1 teaspoon lemon juice
1 tablespoon grapefruit zest
1 tablespoon brown sugar
2 cloves garlic, minced
1½ teaspoons grated fresh ginger
1 teaspoon cumin
1 teaspoon ground coriander

Chicken:
4 boneless, skinless chicken breast halves cut into 1-inch cubes
8 wooden or metal skewers
Grapefruit dipping sauce (recipe follows)

1. Combine soy, fruit juices, zest, brown sugar, garlic, ginger, cumin and coriander, in a small bowl,

2. Pour marinade over chicken in a large shallow non-reactive baking dish. Marinate overnight in the refrigerator.

3. If using wooden skewers, soak them in water for at least 30 minutes before using them to prevent burning.

4. Prepare gas or charcoal grill for direct grilling.

5. Thread chicken cubes onto skewers.

6. Grill for 4 to 5 minutes per side, turning often. Serve with grapefruit dipping sauce.

Servings: 4 (2 skewers per person)

Grapefruit Dipping Sauce

This dipping sauce can double as a syrup for pancakes, waffles or crumpets.

1 tablespoon cornstarch
Dash salt
Dash cinnamon
¾ cup boiling water
½ cup orange blossom honey
1 teaspoon grapefruit zest
1 teaspoon grapefruit juice

1. Combine cornstarch, salt and cinnamon in a 1-quart saucepan.

2. Add water gradually, stirring well.

3. Add honey, heat to boiling and cook, stirring constantly for 5 minutes or until sauce has thickened.

4. Add a remaining ingredients; cook until heated through.

Yield: About 1 cup

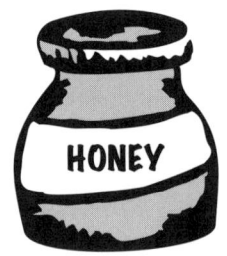

Spicy Grapefruit Chicken Stir-Fry

A successful stir-fry depends on getting all the ingredients ready in advance so that when the fire is hot, and the oil in the pan is sizzling, you can move like lightning.

1 (8-ounce) box vermicelli or rice noodles

Sauce:
½ cup frozen grapefruit juice concentrate, thawed
2 tablespoons grapefruit marmalade
½ cup water
½ teaspoon crushed red pepper flakes
2 teaspoons fresh grated ginger
2 tablespoons soy sauce
2 cloves garlic, minced
2 tablespoons cornstarch
½ teaspoon salt

Stir Fry:
3 tablespoons olive oil (divided use)
1 large green bell pepper, cut in strips
1 large red bell pepper, cut in strips
2 carrots, peeled and sliced diagonally into ½-inch pieces
1 (6-ounce) can sliced water chestnuts, drained
1 teaspoon sesame oil
2 cups boneless, skinless chicken breast cut into 1-inch cubes
½ teaspoon salt

Garnish:
1 teaspoon toasted sesame seeds
1 tablespoon chopped parsley

1. Cook vermicelli or noodles according to package directions.
2. While pasta cooks, make sauce by mixing together juice concentrate, marmalade, water, pepper flakes, ginger, soy and garlic in a small bowl. Combine cornstarch and salt; sprinkle over contents in the bowl. Stir well to incorporate. Set aside.
3. Drain pasta. Keep warm.

Recipe continues on next page ⊃

4. Heat 1½ tablespoons of the olive oil in a large skillet or wok. Add pepper strips, carrots and water chestnuts; stir-fry until crisp tender, about 4 minutes. Remove vegetables from pan with a slotted spoon; set aside.

5. Add to pan the remaining 1½ tablespoons olive oil and sesame oil. Sprinkle chicken with salt; add to the pan. Stir-fry about 5 minutes or until chicken is cooked through.

6. Add reserved sauce to the pan along with vegetables. Cook, stirring until mixture begins to thicken, about 2 minutes.

7. Serve over pasta; garnish with sesame seeds and parsley.

Servings: 4

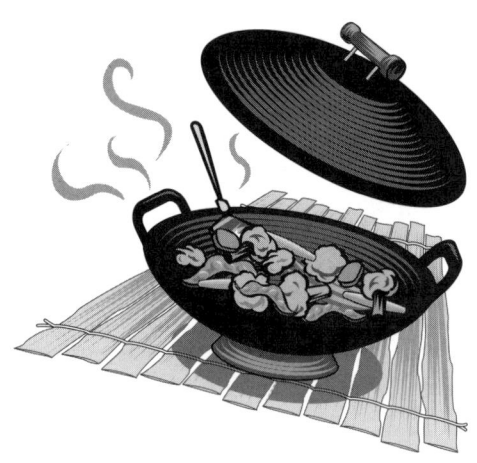

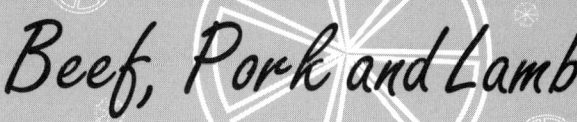

Marinated Steak with Citrus Salsa

This recipe was published some years ago by the Florida Department of Citrus in a cookbook called "Fit, Fresh & Fast" – a wonderful compendium of healthful dishes based on citrus flavors. All were designed to be good to eat and good for you.

¾ cup grapefruit juice concentrate, thawed
1 to 2 jalapeno peppers, seeded and finely chopped
1 teaspoon black pepper
1 teaspoon paprika
½ cup water
1 (1 to 1½ pounds) beef flank steak
¼ cup thinly sliced scallions (white part only)
2 tablespoons snipped fresh flat-leaf parsley
1 tablespoon lime juice
Dash of salt
2 oranges peeled, seeded, and chopped
1 grapefruit, peeled, seeded and chopped
6 (6- to 7-inch) flour tortillas, warmed

1. Combine thawed concentrate, jalapeno, black pepper, and paprika. Reserve 2 tablespoon of the mixture for salsa. Add water to remaining mixture.

2. Score steak by making shallow cuts at 1-inch intervals diagonally across steak in a diamond pattern. Repeat on second side. Place in a plastic bag set in a shallow dish. Pour marinade over steak; close bag. Marinate in the refrigerator for 2 to 24 hours; turn bag occasionally.

3. Meanwhile, in a non-metallic bowl, stir together the reserved 2 tablespoons juice concentrate mixture, scallions, parsley, lime juice and salt. Add chopped oranges and grapefruit; stir gently. Cover and chill at least 30 minutes to blend flavors.

4. Remove meat from bag. Discard marinade. Place steak on an unheated rack of a broiler pan that has been sprayed with non-stick cooking spray.

Recipe continues on next page ⊃

5. Broil 3 inches from heat for 6 minutes. Turn and broil 7 to 8 minutes more for medium-rare.

6. Cut across the grain into thin slices.

Servings: 6

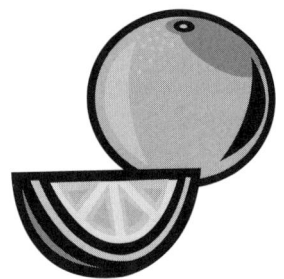

Slow-Cooked Glazed Short Ribs

Short ribs are delicious when long braising and stewing turns the chewy and inexpensive cut of meat into tender morsels. With these Asian-inspired ribs, grapefruit provides all the right flavor notes.

1 sweet onion, cut into wedges
1 red pepper, cut into strips
3 pounds beef short ribs
1 cup grapefruit marmalade
⅓ cup grapefruit juice
2 tablespoons rice vinegar
1 tablespoon soy sauce
2 teaspoons five-spice powder
2 teaspoons grated fresh ginger
½ to 1½ teaspoons chile oil
2 cloves garlic, minced

1. Place onions wedges and pepper strips in a 3½- to 5-quart slow cooker. Add short ribs.

2. Combine marmalade, grapefruit juice, rice vinegar, soy, five-spice powder, ginger, chile oil and garlic in a medium bowl. Reserve ⅔ cup of the marmalade mixture for sauce; cover and chill. Pour the remaining marmalade mixture over ribs, onion and peppers.

3. Cover and cook on low-heat setting for 9 or 10 hours or on high-heat settings for 5½ to 6 hours.

4. To create the sauce, heat reserved marmalade mixture in a small saucepan until boiling. Reduce heat. Simmer uncovered for 5 minutes.

5. Remove short ribs, onions and peppers from the slow cooker; discard cooking liquid. Serve short ribs and vegetables with the sauce.

Servings: 4 to 6.

Wine-Marinated London Broil

Inexpensive London broil benefits from marinating in a heady mix of red wine and grapefruit juice.

½ cup peanut oil
¾ cup soy sauce
2 tablespoons Worcestershire sauce
2 cloves garlic, minced
2 tablespoons dry Chinese mustard
2 tablespoons salt
1 tablespoon ground pepper
1 cup dry red wine
2 teaspoons dried rosemary leaves
½ cup grapefruit juice
1 tablespoon lemon juice
2 pounds London broil

1. Combine all ingredients except the London broil in a quart jar. Cover tightly and shake vigorously. Place London broil in a 13" x 9" x 2" glass or ceramic pan.

2. Pour marinade over the roast. Turn to coat completely. Cover and refrigerate overnight, turning occasionally.

3. Preheat broiler or grill for 10 minutes.

4. Pour off marinade and discard. Place London broil on a grill or broiler rack that has been sprayed with non-stick cooking spray.

5. Broil or grill 3 inches from source of heat for 5 minutes.

6. Turn. Broil 5 more minutes.

7. Remove from grill or broiler and cut across the grain into thin slices.

Servings: 8 to 10.

Glorious Grapefruit Glazed Pork Chops

Sherry vinegar can be found among the many vinegars on super-market shelves. It gives a sweet tang to this appealing glaze.

1 tablespoon vegetable oil
4 pork chops, about ¾-inch thick
Salt and pepper
2 tablespoons grapefruit marmalade
½ cup grapefruit juice
1 tablespoon sherry vinegar

1. Heat oil in a 10" skillet over medium-high heat.

2. Add chops, brown on both sides, seasoning with salt and pepper, about five minutes. Drain off excess fat.

3. Combine marmalade, grapefruit juice and vinegar in a small bowl, mixing well. Pour over chops. Cover, simmer 30 minutes or until chops are done.

4. Remove chops to a warm platter.

5. Bring sauce to boiling; cook until slightly thickened, about five minutes.

6. Spoon over chops just before serving.

Servings: 4

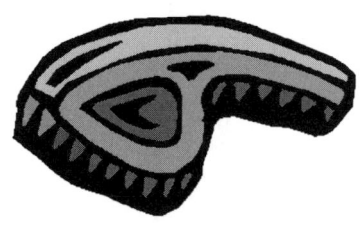

Sun Ray Oven Barbecued Ribs

There are days when you won't want to light up the grill, but that doesn't mean you can't enjoy wonderful outdoor flavor. It can be captured in the kitchen oven.

½ **cup butter**
¾ **cup finely chopped onions**
¾ **cup catsup**
⅓ **cup grapefruit juice**
3 **tablespoons dark brown sugar**
3 **tablespoons Worcestershire sauce**
2 **tablespoons prepared mustard**
1 **teaspoon salt**
Black pepper to taste
¾ **cup water**
2 **pounds country-style pork spare ribs**

1. Preheat oven to 350 degrees F.
2. Melt butter over medium heat in a 10" skillet. Add onion and sauté for 5 minutes.
3. Combine catsup, grapefruit juice, sugar, Worcestershire sauce, mustard, salt, pepper and water in a large glass bowl; add to pan and simmer for 15 minutes, stirring once or twice.
4. Place ribs in a 13" x 9" x 2" glass or ceramic roasting dish; pour sauce over the ribs.
5. Roast for 1½ to 2 hours, basting and turning occasionally.

Servings: 6

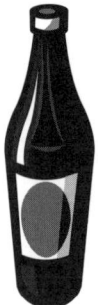

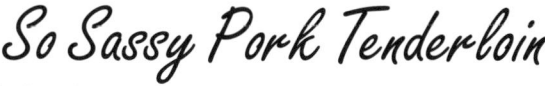

So Sassy Pork Tenderloin

Pork tenderloin has many health benefits, but its luscious taste is still the best reason to enjoy. The marinade is an unlikely combination of wine, celery and juice that lends an unforgettable taste.

1½ pounds boneless pork tenderloin

Marinade:
1 cup dry white wine
Stalk of celery, minced
¼ cup grapefruit juice

Rub:
1 tablespoon crushed capers
**2 teaspoons fresh rosemary or 1 teaspoon dried
    rosemary**
⅛ teaspoon freshly ground black pepper

Garnish:
Grapefruit wedges

1. Trim fat from tenderloin; discard. Place roast in a 13" x 9" x 2" glass or ceramic baking dish.
2. Combine water, celery, and grapefruit juice. Pour over the roast, turning once or twice to coat. Cover and refrigerate for 30 minutes.
3. Preheat oven to 350 degrees F.
4. Combine capers, rosemary and black pepper. Set aside.
5. Remove roast from the refrigerator. Turn in the marinade to coat all sides.
6. Pour off marinade and discard.
7. Rub dry mixture over tenderloin.
8. Roast uncovered 1 hour or until thermometer inserted in the thickest part of the tenderloin registers 170 degrees F.
9. Remove from oven; cover with foil. Allow to stand 10 minutes before serving.
10. Garnish with grapefruit wedges.

Servings: 8

Sunny Funny Ham Kabobs

Wait until you taste the heat from grapefruit, honey and mustard. It fairly sparkles on your palate — all sweet, tart and crisp.

Store-bought honey-mustard barbecue sauce
½ cup grapefruit marmalade
24 1" ham cubes
1 small grapefruit cut into six wedges

1. Prepare gas or charcoal grill for cooking.
2. Combine sauce and marmalade in a small bowl; mix well. Remove ½ cup of the mixture for basting; reserve remaining mixture.
3. Cut grapefruit wedges in half.
4. Thread ham and grapefruit wedges alternately on skewers.
5. Brush with ½ cup barbecue sauce mixture reserved for basting.
6. Grill over medium-hot coals or medium-high grill for 10 minutes or until browned, turning frequently and basting with remaining barbecue mixture. Serve with reserved sauce mixture.

Servings: 6

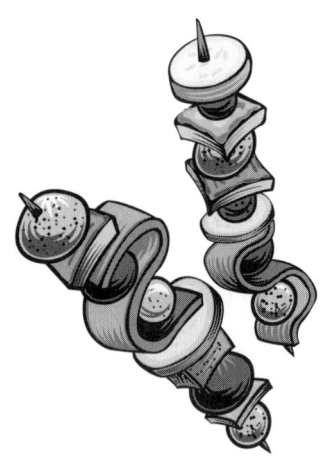

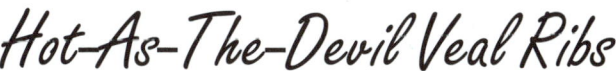

Hot-As-The-Devil Veal Ribs

The fresh red chile lends fire and color to this dish. The grapefruit provides a cooling, mellowing element.

4 pounds breast of veal
1 teaspoon salt
Dash pepper
1 teaspoon garlic salt
½ cup chopped onion
½ cup diced celery
1 fresh red chile, seeded and chopped finely
¼ cup grapefruit juice
¼ cup honey-mustard barbecue sauce
¼ cup sunflower oil
1 cup breadcrumbs

1. Separate ribs. Place in a single layer in a 13" x 9" x 2" glass or ceramic baking dish.

2. Sprinkle seasoning, onion, celery and red chile on top. Cover and bake at 325 degrees F. for 2 hours.

3. Combine grapefruit juice, honey-mustard and oil. Set aside.

4. Remove meat and drain some of the liquid pan juices. Spread reserved dressing over ribs. Pat on breadcrumbs, coating uniformly and thoroughly. Bake ½ hour longer, uncovered, at 400 degrees.

Servings: 8

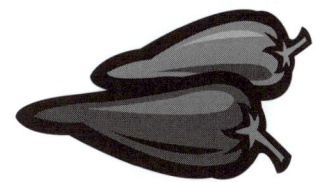

Grilled Marmaladed Marinated Lamb Chops

The lamb chops are tenderized in a slightly sweet, yet sharp grapefruit-flavored marinade that has been spiked with fresh ginger.

2 tablespoons grapefruit marmalade
1 teaspoon fresh ginger
1 garlic clove, finely chopped
¼ cup white wine vinegar
¼ cup grapefruit juice
¼ cup lemon juice
½ cup olive oil
Freshly ground black pepper
8 rib lamb chops (1½ pounds total)

1. Put marmalade, ginger, garlic, wine vinegar and fruit juices in a 1-quart non-reactive saucepan over medium heat, stirring, until marmalade has melted.

2. Simmer until reduced to 1 cup. Pour into a bowl to cool.

3. Stir in oil and season with black pepper to taste.

4. Pour into a sealable plastic bag. Add lamb chops, then seal bag, pressing out excess air and turning to distribute marinade. Marinate lamb, chilled, turning occasionally, at least 1 hour.

5. Prepare gas or charcoal grill for cooking. If using a charcoal grill, open vents on bottom of grill and on lid.

6. Remove lamb from marinade; discard marinade. When fire or gas grill is medium hot, grill lamb on lightly oiled grill rack, turning once, about 4 minutes for medium-rare. Transfer to a platter.

Servings: 4

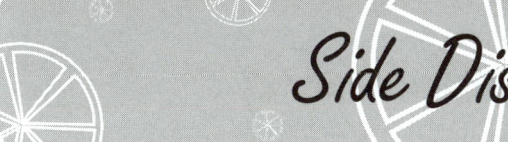
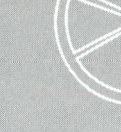
Fruited Couscous

The ancient Middle Eastern dish of couscous is one of the quickest and easiest side dishes available to the modern cook. This adapted recipe, developed for Tropicana Pure Premium, the citrus fruit juice company founded in Florida back in 1947, makes an appealing side dish for a seafood, lamb or poultry entrée.

1 cup grapefruit juice
2 teaspoons extra virgin olive oil
½ teaspoon ground cinnamon
½ teaspoon ground coriander
¼ teaspoon salt
⅛ teaspoon cayenne pepper (optional)
½ cup dried fruit bits (see Note 1)
¾ cup boxed couscous mix (see Note 2)
¼ cup toasted slivered almonds

1. Combine juice, olive oil, cinnamon, coriander, salt and, if desired, cayenne pepper in 1½-quart saucepan; mix well.

2. Stir in fruit. Cover and bring to a boil.

3. Stir in couscous. Cover and remove from heat. Let stand 5 minutes.

4. Gently fluff couscous with fork. Sprinkle with almonds. Serve immediately.

Servings: 4

Note 1: Raisins, dried cranberries or any combination of dried fruits, chopped, may be substituted for dried fruit bits.

Note 2: Couscous may be prepared in the microwave oven. Combine juice, olive oil, cinnamon, coriander and cayenne pepper in 1½-quart microwaveable casserole with lid; mix well. Stir in fruit. Cover. Microwave on HIGH until boiling, about 4 minutes. Uncover; stir in couscous. Cover tightly. Let stand 5 minutes. Fluff with fork.

Citrus Mashed Parsnips

Grapefruit juice brings out the natural sweetness of parsnips in this pretty vegetable side dish.

1 pound peeled parsnips, cut into bite size pieces
1 tablespoons butter
⅓ cup grapefruit juice
¼ teaspoon grapefruit zest
Pinch of cinnamon
Pinch of nutmeg
1 teaspoon turbinado or brown sugar (see Note)

1. Place parsnips in a 2-quart saucepan with enough water to cover. Bring to a boil; lower heat and continue to simmer over medium-high heat for about 12 minutes. Drain.

2. Add butter, juice, zest, cinnamon, nutmeg and sugar. Mash together.

Servings: 4

Note: *Turbinado sugar is a less processed cane sugar. It can be found in supermarkets.*

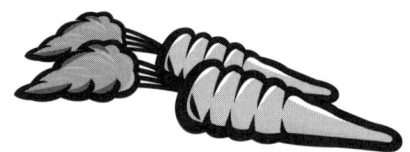

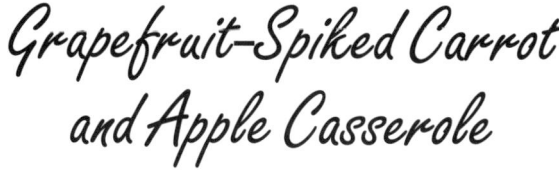

Grapefruit-Spiked Carrot and Apple Casserole

No matter where you are, apples and carrots signify the coming of fall. You can whip up this harvest time side dish in no time at all to enjoy these great Florida flavors!

5 tablespoons sugar
2 tablespoons flour
¼ cup melted butter
¾ cup grapefruit juice at room temperature
5 apples peeled, cored and sliced thin
2 cups peeled, cooked carrots

1. Preheat oven to 350 degrees F.

2. Combine sugar and flour in a medium mixing bowl. Stir in melted butter and grapefruit juice, stirring well to combine.

3. Layer apples and carrots in a greased 1½-quart shallow casserole dish. Pour juice mixture over top.

4. Bake for 45 minutes.

Servings: 4 to 6

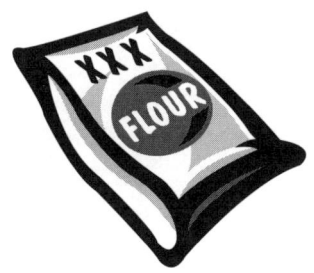

Ruby Red Beets

The tanginess of grapefruit and the natural sweetness of beets pair well in this fruit-vegetable combination.

1 tablespoons cornstarch
2 tablespoons sugar
½ teaspoon salt
1 cup Ruby Red grapefruit juice
1 tablespoon grapefruit zest
2 tablespoons butter
1 (16-ounce) can beets, drained

1. Combine cornstarch, sugar and salt in a 2-quart saucepan. Add grapefruit juice and zest.

2. Heat slowly over low heat, stirring until thickened. Stir in butter in small pieces.

3. Add beets; heat through.

Servings: 4

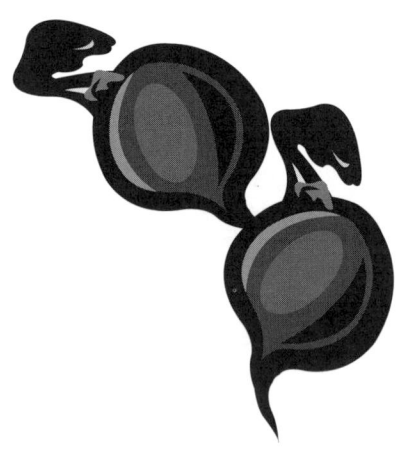

Butternut Puree with Grapefruit

Butternuts are very big squash, but don't be daunted. Use a very sharp knife to slice as deeply as you can, then give the squash a good, hard smash on the countertop. It should break open. Remove the seeds and peel the pieces. The results are worth the work.

3½ pounds butternut squash, peeled, seeded and cut into 2-inch chunks
¼ cup extra virgin olive oil
2 to 3 tablespoons grapefruit juice
Salt and pepper, to taste
Cinnamon

1. Steam butternut chunks for 15 to 20 minutes until very tender. Reserve steaming liquid.

2. Press squash through a ricer or food mill set over a large bowl.

3. Stir in olive oil, grapefruit juice and enough of the reserved liquid to reach desired consistency.

4. Season with salt and pepper. Dust with cinnamon before serving.

Servings: 10

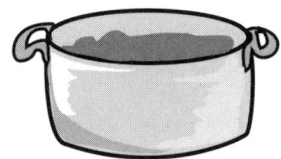

Grapefruit Baked Sweet Potatoes

Try this as a nice alternative to the cloyingly sweet marshmallow-topped baked sweet potatoes that show up on holiday tables.

2 (1-pound, 2-ounce) cans sweet potatoes, drained
1 small, thin-skinned, unpeeled seedless grapefruit
¼ cup butter
½ cup firmly packed brown sugar
¼ teaspoon salt
Dash cinnamon
Dash ginger

1. Preheat oven to 350 degrees F.

2. Slice sweet potatoes into a 9" x 9" x 2" baking dish.

3. Cut grapefruit into chunks.

4. Working in two batches, place half of grapefruit and half of remaining ingredients into a food processor. Process until smooth.

5. Combine the two batches and spoon over baked potatoes.

6. Bake for 30 minutes.

Servings: 6 to 8

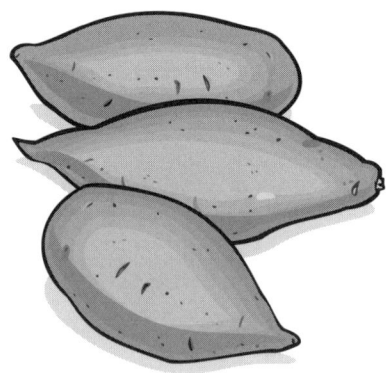

Sun Glazed Roasted Pumpkin

This is a lovely fall dish that can be made only during the all too brief time when fresh pumpkin is in the market. It has a unique sweet and sour flavor.

2 pounds pumpkin (whole or in pieces)
¼ cup butter, melted
¼ cup turbinado sugar (see Note)
½ teaspoon ground ginger
⅛ teaspoon salt
⅛ teaspoon ground black pepper
3 tablespoons grapefruit marmalade
1 tablespoon room temperature grapefruit juice

1. Preheat oven to 350 degrees F.

2. If using a whole pumpkin, cut the pumpkin in half, remove and discard seeds and fibers. Peel pumpkin and cut into 1½-inch cubes. Set aside.

3. Combine melted butter, sugar, ginger, salt, pepper and marmalade. Toss with pumpkin cubes.

4. Turn into a buttered 8" × 8" × 2" baking dish. Sprinkle with grapefruit juice. Cover and bake for 45 minutes.

5. Remove cover and bake 30 minutes more or until pumpkin is tender, basting frequently with pan juices.

Servings: 6

Note: Turbinado sugar is a less refined sugar widely available in supermarkets.

Corn Fritters with Sunset Sauce

Many restaurants in Florida bring corn fritters to the table first thing. Dusted with powdered sugar and bearing a beautiful golden crust, they are irresistible. Problem is, you could fill your tummy before the appetizers arrive.

Sunset Sauce:
1 (6-ounce) can frozen grapefruit juice concentrate, thawed
1 ¼ cups water
2 tablespoons cornstarch
1 tablespoon butter

Fritters:
1 cup flour
1 teaspoon baking powder
1 teaspoon salt
Dash pepper
1 cup cream-style corn
2 eggs
Vegetable oil for frying

1. Combine concentrate with water. Add 1 tablespoon of the mixture to the cornstarch to make a thick paste.

2. Add the paste to the reconstituted juice in a 2-quart saucepan. Cook and stir over low heat until smooth, clear and slightly thick.

3. Stir in butter, until melted and mixture is shiny. Set aside.

4. To create the fritters, combine flour and baking powder, salt and pepper in a large mixing bowl. Add cream-style corn and mix well.

5. In another small bowl, beat eggs until they are light and frothy. Add to corn-flour mixture, incorporating well.

6. Heat oil in a deep pan or deep fat fryer until temperature is 370 degrees F.

7. Carefully drop teaspoonsful of the mixture into the hot fat and fry until golden brown. Drain on paper towels. Serve hot with grapefruit sauce on the side.

Servings: 4

Sauces & Condiments

Grapefruit Butter Sauce

Bruno's in Destin and Gulf Breeze, Fla., offer consumers delicious recipes at www.brunos.com. This versatile and easy-to-make grapefruit butter sauce is a nice accompaniment to seafood and poultry.

1½ cups fresh grapefruit juice (divided use)
1 cup sugar
1 teaspoon grapefruit zest
¼ cup white wine vinegar
1 tablespoon shallots, minced
¼ cup heavy cream
2 sticks butter, cut into pieces
Salt and pepper to taste

1. Combine 1 cup grapefruit juice, sugar and zest in a 2-quart saucepan.

2. Cook over medium heat, stirring occasionally, until reduced to a thick syrup. Set aside.

3. In another saucepan, combine the remaining grapefruit juice, vinegar and shallots. Simmer until reduced by half.

4. Add the heavy cream and cook for 1 minute. Lower heat and gradually whisk in the butter, 1 tablespoon at a time.

5. Remove from heat. Add the thick grapefruit syrup, salt and pepper; stir gently to combine.

Yield: About 2 cups

Grapefruit Grove Sauce

The citrusy taste of the buttery sauce adds a whole new flavor dimension when spooned over fish or vegetables.

4 tablespoons sesame seeds
¼ cup butter
2 tablespoons grapefruit juice

1. Toast sesame seeds in a 7" frying pan over low heat, watching carefully as the seeds burn easily. When seeds are fragrant and light brown in color, add the butter, stirring until melted.

2. Add the grapefruit juice; stir to combine. Heat through.

Yield: about ½ cup

Grapefruit-Spiked Barbecue Sauce

This is a lighter barbecue sauce that goes well with fin- or shellfish, bringing out a delicate briny flavor instead of masking it.

1 teaspoon dry mustard
1 tablespoon water
2 tablespoons grapefruit juice
1 tablespoon lemon juice
2 tablespoons apple cider vinegar
1 teaspoon coarse grain sea salt
½ teaspoon garlic salt
½ teaspoon paprika
½ teaspoon fresh-ground black pepper
¼ teaspoon cayenne

1. Combine dry mustard and water, mixing well.

2. Add to remaining ingredients in a 1-quart saucepan over medium heat, stirring well to combine. Bring to a simmer (do not boil).

3. Remove from heat.

4. Brush mixture over grilled fish or shellfish.

Yield: about a ½ cup

Grapefruit Compound Butter

Compound butters (beurres composes) are mixtures of butter with other ingredients such as herbs, cheeses and spices. What goes into them is a matter of taste, but try this one with grapefruit juice, pepper and parsley over corn on the cob or steamed vegetables.

⅔ cup butter, softened
⅓ cup chopped fresh flat-leaf parsley
2 teaspoons salt
½ teaspoon fresh ground black pepper
¼ teaspoon paprika
¼ cup grapefruit juice

1. Blend butter with remaining ingredients.

2. Place in a small mold or bowl. Cover and refrigerate.

Yield: about ¼ cup

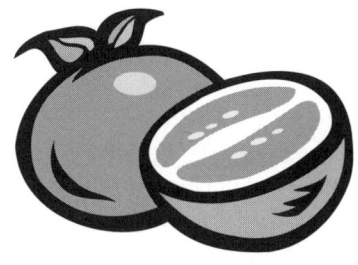

Florida Barbecue Sauce

Floridians adore barbecue sauce and developed a special style all their own that has a slightly vinegary, less sweet taste. This recipe is an expansion of that with grapefruit thrown into the mix with wonderful effect.

4 teaspoons dry mustard
¼ cup water
4 pounds diced, fresh tomatoes
½ cup chopped onion
2 cloves garlic, chopped
1 cup grapefruit juice
⅔ cup apple cider vinegar
⅓ cup lemon juice
1 tablespoons salt
4 teaspoons paprika
2 teaspoons cayenne
2 tablespoons datil pepper sauce or other bottled red-hot sauce such as Frank's Red Hot Sauce (see Note)

1. Combine mustard and water. Set aside

2. In a 3-quart saucepan or Dutch oven, cook tomatoes, onion and garlic over low heat for about 25 minutes stirring occasionally to avoid burning.

3. Press mixture through a sieve back into the saucepan or Dutch oven. Discard pulp.

4. Add mustard-water mixture along with remaining ingredients. Heat to boiling over medium-high heat. Lower heat and simmer to desired consistency.

5. Ladle into three 1-pint containers. Refrigerate. Sauce will keep for about 3 weeks. Reheat with a little butter, and brush over meats or poultry during the last stages of barbecuing. Or serve on the side.

Yield: about three pints

Note: Datil pepper sauce is a fiery condiment that historians believe was brought to St. Augustine by Minorcan settlers in the 1700's.

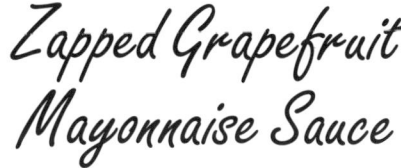

Zapped Grapefruit Mayonnaise Sauce

Thank the microwave for being so handy. This sauce comes together in a matter of seconds, and brings out the best in fresh seafood.

2 tablespoons white grapefruit juice
Dash of ground white pepper
½ cup mayonnaise

1. Combine all ingredients, stirring well.

2. Heat in a microwave-safe dish for 35 seconds on HIGH. Stir. Serve over fish.

Yield: about a ½ cup

Grapefruit-Tarragon Sauce

Tarragon has an aroma reminiscent of anise. It pairs beautifully with grapefruit juice in this easy-to-make sauce that can be served over-chilled chicken, shrimp or sliced tomatoes.

½ cup mayonnaise
1 teaspoon chopped fresh tarragon (½ teaspoon dried)
2 teaspoons white grapefruit juice

1. Combine all ingredients in a small bowl. Mix well.

2. Refrigerate until ready to use.

Yield: about a ½ cup

Sunshine Sauce

Dress up vanilla or banana pudding, or a slice of unfrosted cake with this thin, frothy and zesty dessert sauce.

⅔ **cup heavy cream**
¼ **cup butter at room temperature**
1 **cup sifted confectioners' sugar**
1 **large egg yolk**
¼ **cup grapefruit juice**
¼ **teaspoon grapefruit zest**
¼ **teaspoon cinnamon**

1. Whip heavy cream in a chilled mixing bowl. Refrigerate until ready to use.

2. In another mixing bowl, whip butter until fluffy. Gradually blend in confectioners' sugar, and then beat in egg yolk, grapefruit juice, zest and cinnamon.

3. Fold in whipped cream.

Yield: 1½ cups

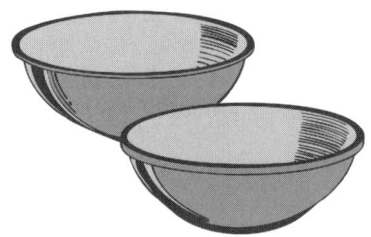

Golden Grapefruit Sauce

A simple dessert sauce, Golden Grapefruit Sauce is light, sweet and slightly tart. Serve over warm pudding or toasted pound cake.

½ **cup sugar**
1 **tablespoon cornstarch**
½ **teaspoon salt**
¼ **cup cold water**
¾ **cup boiling water**
1 **large separated egg yolk**
3 **tablespoons white grapefruit juice**
1 **teaspoon grapefruit zest**
2 **tablespoons butter**

1. Combine sugar, cornstarch and salt in a 2-quart saucepan.

2. Add cold water and mix well. Gradually stir in boiling water. Continue to stir and cook over medium heat for 10 to 12 minutes or until clear and medium thickness.

3. Blend separated yolk with grapefruit juice; gradually stir into the heated mixture. Cook 1 minute, stirring constantly.

4. Add zest and butter, stirring until butter has melted and is fully incorporated.

5. Serve warm.

Yield: about 1½ cups

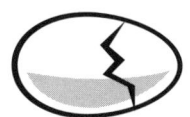

Grapefruit Grove Snack Cake

Grapefruit creates the dominant flavor and color of this light cake with a powerful citrus taste.

Cake:
1 small pink grapefruit
1 cup seedless raisins
½ cup walnuts
2 cups flour
1 teaspoon baking soda
1 cup sugar
1 teaspoon salt
½ cup vegetable shortening such as Crisco®
¾ cup milk
2 eggs
¾ cup milk (divided use)

Topping:
⅓ cup grapefruit juice
⅓ cup sugar
¼ cup chopped walnuts
½ teaspoon cinnamon

1. Preheat oven to 350 degrees F.

2. Prepare a 12" x 8" x 2" baking pan with non-stick baking spray.

3. Halve grapefruit; squeeze to extract juice. You will need ⅓ cup for topping.

4. Chop one of the grapefruit halves with pulp and rind in a food processor along with raisins and walnuts. Process until grapefruit is in ¼-inch pieces.

5. Combine the flour, baking soda, sugar and salt in a large mixing bowl. Beat in shortening and ½ cup of the milk on low until well combined.

6. Beat on high speed for 2 minutes.

Recipe continues on next page ⊃

Grapefruit Grove Snack Cake

7. Add eggs and remaining ¼ cup of milk. Fold grapefruit-raisin mixture into the batter. Pour into the prepared pan and bake for 40 to 50 minutes.

8. Cool on a rack for 10 minutes. Remove from pan and finish cooling on the rack. While cake is still warm, drizzle grapefruit juice over the top.

9. Combine ⅓ cup of sugar with walnuts and cinnamon. Sprinkle over the cake.

Yield: one 12" x 8" cake.

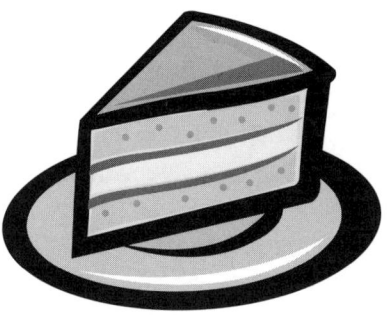

Grapefruit Cake Custard

This is a citrusy take on old-fashioned "spoon bread." The cake's texture is so moist it's almost a pudding! The taste is soft and mellow except for the lovely little spike from the grapefruit's natural sweet but tart flavor.

1 cup sugar
1 tablespoon butter
2 egg yolks
3 tablespoons grapefruit juice
¼ cup flour
1 cup milk
2 egg whites
Pinch of salt
Non-dairy whipped topping for garnish
Candied grapefruit zest (recipe follows)

1. Preheat oven to 350 degrees F.
2. Cream together sugar and butter with an electric mixer in a medium-size mixing bowl. Beat until smooth and lemon colored.
3. Add egg yolks and beat well.
4. Add grapefruit juice, flour and then, milk.
5. Clean beaters. Any oil or egg yolk residue will prevent whites from whipping.
6. Whip egg whites with salt in another mixing bowl until stiff and shiny. Fold into batter.
7. Pour into a 9"-round baking pan that has been sprayed with non-stick baking spray.
8. Place baking pan in a larger baking pan filled with water. Bake for about 30 minutes or until cake pulls away from the edge of the pan.
9. Cool for about 10 minutes.
10. Serve warm or chilled with whipped dairy topping and candied grapefruit zest.

Servings: 6 to 8

Candied Grapefruit Zest

This is an old-time recipe that needs to be resurrected. The tartness of the citrus peel and the sweetness of the sugar make an irresistible combination.

2 brightly colored grapefruit
⅔ cup granulated sugar
Grapefruit juice as needed

1. Remove the colored part of the grapefruit rind using a small knife or zester.

2. Cut peel into ¼-inch wide strips enough to measure 6 tablespoons full.

3. Squeeze the juice out of the peeled grapefruit, adding more if needed to measure 1½ cups.

4. Place the peel in a small non-reactive saucepan and cover with 1 inch of water. Bring to a boil, reduce the heat to medium and simmer uncovered for about 5 minutes.

5. Drain in a small sieve and discard the liquid. Return the peel to the saucepan along with the sugar and juice. Bring to a boil, stirring to dissolve the sugar, and then reduce heat to medium-low. Simmer, uncovered, until the peel is translucent and the syrup is thickened, about 7 minutes.

6. Remove from the heat. If the syrup is too thick, stir in a teaspoon or more of grapefruit juice.

7. Refrigerate for up to 2 days. Return to room temperature to use.

Yield: about 1 cup

Indian River Grapefruit Meringue Cake

This recipe from Mary Cummings of New Smyrna Beach was the grand prizewinner in the Fresh Start Recipe Contest sponsored by Florida Citrus Growers. It is a light dessert with fabulous grapefruit flavor in each of its three layers.

Cake:
1½ large fresh grapefruit
¼ cup butter
½ cup sugar
2 egg yolks (reserve whites at room temperature)
1 whole egg
1 cup all-purpose flour
1 teaspoon baking powder
1 teaspoon grapefruit zest
¼ cup whole milk
2 tablespoons grapefruit juice
½ teaspoon vanilla

Filling:
2 eggs, separated (add whites to reserved whites in bowl)
1 cup water
¾ cup sugar
⅓ cup all-purpose flour
1 teaspoon grapefruit zest
⅓ cup grapefruit juice
1 tablespoon butter

Topping:
Reserved egg whites
½ teaspoon cream of tartar
½ cup sugar combined with 1 teaspoon grapefruit zest
Sprig of fresh mint

1. Grease and flour a 9" round cake pan.

2. Preheat oven to 350 degrees F.

3. Grate rind of one grapefruit to measure 1 tablespoon zest.

Recipe continues on next page ⊃

Indian River Grapefruit Meringue Cake

4. Squeeze same grapefruit to yield ½ cup unstrained juice.

5. Cut grapefruit half into segments. Reserve all separately.

6. To create the cake: Cream butter with an electric mixer set on medium speed. Gradually stir in sugar until fluffy.

7. Add 2 egg yolks and whole egg; beat well.

8. Combine flour, baking powder, and zest, and then add alternately with milk and juice to the butter mixture, beginning and ending with flour mixture and beating well after each addition.

9. Stir in vanilla.

10. Pour batter into prepared pan. Bake for 28 to 30 minutes or until toothpick inserted in center tests clean.

11. Cool in pan 10 minutes, then remove from pan to cool completely.

12. To create the filling: Combine egg yolks and water in a small bowl.

13. Combine sugar and flour in a heavy saucepan; add yolk mixture and zest.

14. Cook over medium heat, stirring until mixture thickens and boils.

15. Remove from heat; stir in juice and butter. Cover loosely and cool.

16. Place cooled cake on baking sheet. Spoon filling evenly on cake to within ½-inch of edges.

17. To create the topping: Beat the four egg whites (at room temperature) with cream of tartar for 1 minute on high speed in a large mixing bowl.

18. Gradually add sugar/grapefruit zest mixture, beating until stiff peaks form, about 3 minutes.

19. Spread topping over cake filling, covering completely.

20. Form decorative swirls from center to edges using back of tablespoon.

21. Bake for 12 to 15 minutes or until peaks are lightly browned.

22. Cool completely. Just before serving, decorate center top with reserved, well-drained grapefruit segments and a sprig of fresh mint.

Servings: 8

Grapefruit Chiffon Pie
in Walnut Crust

If you are going to bake a pie, make it this one. The unique crust and the citrusy filling make it memorable.

Baked Walnut Pie Shell:
1 cup all-purpose flour
½ teaspoon salt
⅓ cup shortening
¼ cup walnuts, finely chopped
3 to 4 tablespoons cold water

Filling:
1 tablespoon unflavored gelatin
¼ cup water
4 egg yolks
1 cup sugar
½ cup grapefruit juice
1 teaspoon grapefruit zest
4 egg whites

Topping:
1 cup whipping cream
¼ cup sugar
1 teaspoon vanilla extract

1. Preheat oven to 425 degrees F.

2. Combine flour, and salt in a large mixing bowl.

3. Cut in the shortening until particles are the size of small peas.

4. Add walnuts; mix well.

5. Sprinkle cold water over mixture, tossing lightly with fork until dough is moist enough to hold together. Form into a ball.

6. Roll out pastry on a floured pastry cloth to a circle 1½ inches larger than an inverted 9"-pie pan. Fit pastry loosely into pan.

7. Fold edge to form a standing rim; flute. Prick crust with a fork.

8. Bake for 10 to 12 minutes. Remove from oven; cool.

Recipe continues on next page ⊃

9. To create the filling: Soften the gelatin in the cold water. Set aside.

10. While gelatin softens, beat egg yolks. Add half the sugar, grapefruit juice and zest. Continue to beat until very light.

11. Place in a saucepan over very low heat or in a double boiler. Stir until custard consistency is reached. Stir in gelatin. Remove from heat. Cool to room temperature.

12. In a medium-size mixing bowl, beat egg whites, adding in remaining sugar slowly. Fold into gelatin mixture. Pour into pie shell. Chill.

13. Before serving, whip together whipping cream and sugar. Spread over grapefruit filling covering surface completely.

Servings: 6

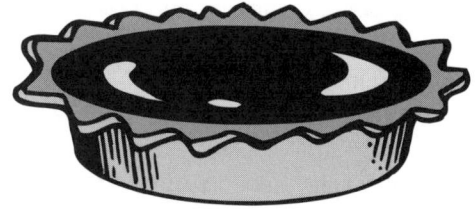

Florida Flower Cake

This is an old-time Florida recipe that was very popular in the 1930s and early 1940s. It can be made with oranges, grapefruit or a combination of both. Decorate simply with citrus segments arranged in a flower pattern. It is a gorgeous cake to set before company.

2½ cups cake flour
1½ teaspoons baking powder
¼ teaspoon salt
1 cup sugar
1 teaspoon grapefruit zest
½ cup shortening
2 eggs
½ cup grapefruit juice

Topping and Filling:
1 cup whipping cream
¼ cup sugar
1 teaspoon vanilla extract
At least 2 dozen grapefruit segments, membranes and all pith removed

1. Preheat oven to 350 degrees F.
2. Spray two 8" or 9" round baking pans with non-stick baking spray.
3. In a large mixing bowl, combine flour, baking powder and salt. Set aside.
4. Add zest to shortening and cream by thoroughly beating with a hand mixer or a whisk until the shortening and zest are light and fluffy.
5. Add eggs, one at a time, beating thoroughly after each addition.
6. Add flour mixture and grapefruit juice alternately in small amounts, beating thoroughly after each addition.
7. Pour into prepared pans. Bake for 30 minutes. Cool for 10 minutes. Remove from pans and completely on a baking rack.

Recipe continues on next page ⟳

8. When cakes are ready to be frosted, whip cream until light and fluffy, then gradually beat in sugar and vanilla. Refrigerate.

9. Place one of the cake layers on a serving dish. Cover the top with grapefruit segments. Cover the segments with whipped cream.

10. Place second layer on top. Cover top with remaining whipped cream, then arrange grapefruit segments in a flower or spoke design. Cake can be served with additional whipped cream on the side.

Yield: One 8- or 9-inch layer cake

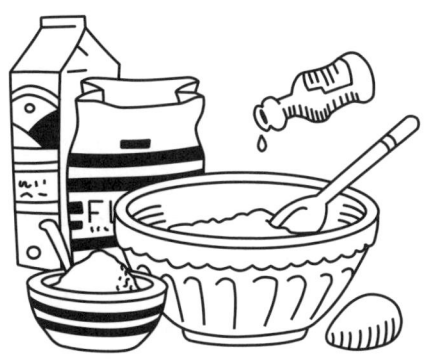

Grapefruit Cake

Devil's food cake is a much-loved American classic. This variation made with grapefruit juice is sinfully good.

Cake:
2 cups light brown sugar (divided use)
1 cup cocoa (divided use)
1½ cups grapefruit juice (divided use)
2 cups cake flour
½ teaspoon baking powder
1 teaspoon baking soda
¼ cup shortening
2 eggs, separated

Frosting:
1 (8-ounce) package softened cream cheese
1 (14-ounce) can sweetened condensed milk
⅓ cup grapefruit juice
1 teaspoon vanilla

1. Preheat oven to 350 degrees F.
2. Spray two 8" layer cake pans with non-stick baking spray.
3. Combine 1 cup light brown sugar, cocoa and 1 cup of the grapefruit juice in a 2-quart saucepan. Cook over medium-high heat until thickened, stirring constantly. Remove pan from the stove. Set aside to cool.
4. Combine flour, baking powder and soda in a large mixing bowl,
5. Cream shortening with remaining cup of sugar in another mixing bowl by beating with a hand mixer or a whisk until light and fluffy.
6. Beat eggs with a fork; add to shortening and beat thoroughly.
7. Add dry ingredients and remaining grapefruit juice alternately in small amounts, beating well after each addition.
8. Fold in cooled brown sugar and cocoa mixture until thoroughly blended.
9. Beat egg whites until stiff. Gently fold into batter.

Recipe continues on next page ⊃

10. Pour into pans and bake for 30 to 35 minutes. Cool for 10 minutes; invert pans onto a cooling rack and carefully lift up and off the cakes. Cool completely.

11. To make the frosting, beat cream cheese in a large mixing bowl, until fluffy; add condensed milk slowly while continuing to beat.

12. Add grapefruit juice and vanilla, beating until smooth.

13. Frost cake with the cream cheese mixture (frosting will set as the cake stands). Refrigerate

Yield: One 8" layer cake

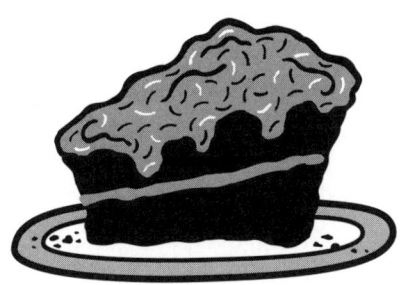

Sunshine Pie

The secret to success is slicing the grapefruit paper-thin. Slices are then baked into the delicate and creamy custard filling.

Favorite pie crust recipe or prepared crusts for an 8-inch double-crust pie
1 egg white mixed with 1 teaspoon water
2 teaspoons sugar
½ teaspoon cinnamon

Filling:
1¼ cup sugar
2 tablespoons flour
⅛ teaspoon salt
¼ cup butter, softened
3 eggs, well beaten
1 small grapefruit
½ cup water
1 teaspoon grapefruit zest

1. Preheat oven to 400 degrees F.

2. Loosely fit bottom crust in an 8" pie pan. Set aside.

3. Prepare grapefruit filling by combining sugar, flour and salt in a large mixing bowl. Blend in softened butter; mix thoroughly with a spoon.

4. Add eggs, blend well until smooth.

5. Peel the grapefruit and remove pith. Cut into paper-thin slices (you'll need about ⅓ cup of grapefruit slices). Set aside.

6. Add water, grapefruit slices and zest to filling mixture. Toss well. Turn into pie pan.

7. Cover with top crust.

8. Fold edge of top crust under lower crust; seal and flute edge.

9. Brush with egg white.

10. Combine sugar and cinnamon, and then sprinkle over pie crust.

11. Cut slits in top crust to allow steam to escape.

12. Bake for 30 to 35 minutes.

Yield: 1 8" pie that can be cut into 6 to 8 servings

Golden Nuggets

These cookies are as bright and sunny as a day at the beach. A tangy, grapefruit-flavored icing tops these easy-to-make moist drop cookies.

Cookies:
2 cups flour
1½ teaspoons baking powder
¼ teaspoon salt
¾ cup shortening
½ cup sugar
¼ cup firmly packed light brown sugar
1 egg, well beaten
2 (2.5 ounce) jars baby food carrots
1 teaspoon vanilla extract
1 cup walnuts, chopped

Grapefruit Icing:
1 cup confectioners' sugar
2 teaspoons grapefruit zest
2 tablespoons grapefruit juice

1. Preheat oven to 400 degrees F.

2. Combine flour, baking powder and salt in a large mixing bowl.

3. Blend together shortening, sugar and light brown sugar, in another mixing bowl, beating well with a mixer or whisk until light and fluffy.

4. Add egg, and then beat well to combine.

5. Blend in dry ingredients in small batches alternately with baby food carrots.

6. Add vanilla. Mix thoroughly. Stir in walnuts. Mix well.

7. Drop by rounded teaspoonsful onto a greased baking sheet. Bake for 12 to15 minutes. Frost while warm.

8. To make frosting: Combine confectioners' sugar, zest and juice. Mix until smooth.

Yield: 5 dozen cookies

Grapefruit Corn Flake Chews

These yummy treats are easy to make and keep quite well. With grapefruit at its height during the winter months, you might find that these chews easily find a place on holiday cookie platters.

1 (14-ounce) can sweetened condensed milk
1 tablespoon grapefruit zest
1 tablespoon grapefruit juice
3½ cups corn flakes, crushed
1⅓ cups shredded coconut
¼ teaspoon salt

1. Preheat oven to 350 degrees F.

2. Combine sweetened condensed milk, zest, grapefruit juice and corn flake crumbs.

3. Add coconut and salt. Let stand about 3 minutes.

4. Drop by teaspoonsful onto greased baking sheet. Bake about 15 minutes.

5. Remove at once from baking sheet.

Yield: About 3½ dozen

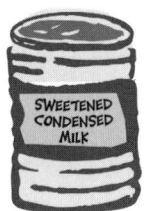

Panna Cotta with Citrus Salad

Royal Caribbean International cruise line, based in Miami, boasts world-renowned galleys. Among the wondrous dishes served is this light and refreshing cooler that can be offered to your guests as a salad or a dessert.

Panna Cotta:
1 tablespoon unflavored gelatin
3 egg whites
½ pint heavy cream, whipped
¼ cup sugar
½ teaspoon lemon zest
½ teaspoon grapefruit zest
½ teaspoon orange zest
1 cinnamon stick
¾ cup buttermilk

Sauce:
1 tablespoon Grand Marnier®
¾ cup freshly squeezed orange juice
¼ cup grapefruit juice
½ teaspoon lemon zest
½ teaspoon grapefruit zest
½ teaspoon orange zest
1 tablespoon sugar

Garnish:
1 orange, segmented
1 grapefruit, segmented
2 tablespoons fresh mint julienne

1. To create the panna cotta, place gelatin in a bowl of lukewarm water to soften.

2. Whisk egg whites with an electric mixer in a small bowl until soft peaks form.

Recipe continues on next page ⊃

Panna Cotta with Citrus Salad

3. Warm cream, sugar, citrus zests, and cinnamon stick in a 1-quart saucepan, over low heat. Remove from heat, discard cinnamon stick and fold in gelatin and buttermilk.

4. Cool, stirring occasionally, for 5 minutes.

5. Fold in egg whites and pour into individual molds. Refrigerate for 6 hours.

6. To make the sauce, mix the Marnier, fruit juices, zests and sugar in a small saucepan, and bring to a boil over medium heat. Reduce heat and simmer for 20 minutes, or until juice is reduced by half.

7. Taka panna cotta out of molds by warming sides under hot running water.

8. Place on chilled plates, with sauce spooned around. Garnish with citrus segments and mint.

Servings: 6

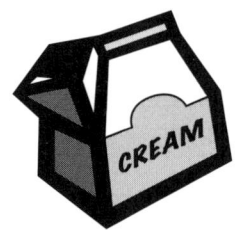

Chocolate Chip Grapefruit Muffins

Muffin lovers will praise the cook for this new twist on a muffin flavor: Grapefruit and chocolate chips. They make for a positively opulent and unexpected breakfast food.

1 small pink grapefruit, washed and dried
1 cup sugar
½ cup butter, softened
2 eggs
½ cup plain yogurt
2 cups flour
1 teaspoon baking powder
½ teaspoon baking soda
½ cup bittersweet chocolate chips

1. Preheat oven to 375 degrees F.

2. Spray a 12-muffin cup baking pan with non-stick baking spray.

3. Grate enough of the grapefruit rind (colored part only) to yield 1 tablespoon of zest. Set aside.

4. Squeeze grapefruit to extract ½ cup juice.

5. Beat sugar and butter in a large bowl until light and fluffy.

6. Add eggs, one at a time, beating well after each addition.

7. Add zest, grapefruit juice and yogurt; mix well. Batter should be quite thin.

8. Combine flour, baking powder and baking soda in a large mixing bowl; sprinkle over liquid mixture along with chocolate chips. Fold in gently, just to blend.

9. Spoon into muffin cups. Bake for 20 to 25 minutes or until golden brown. Serve warm or cool.

Yield: a dozen muffins

Grapefruit Date Nut Bread

The pairing of grapefruit and dates works beautifully in this satisfying bread that can be served at breakfast or as a sweet snack.

1 small grapefruit
1 cup chopped dates (divided use)
1 teaspoon baking soda
1 cup sugar
2 tablespoons butter
1 teaspoon vanilla
1 large egg, beaten
2 cups flour
1 teaspoon baking powder
¼ teaspoon salt
½ cup chopped walnuts

Grapefruit Glaze:
1 cup confectioners' sugar
¼ cup grapefruit juice
1 teaspoon grapefruit zest

1. Preheat oven to 350 degrees F.

2. Squeeze juice from grapefruit into a measuring cup. Fill with boiling water to measure 1 cup.

3. Cut one half of the grapefruit into chunks, then add to a food processor bowl or blender along with ½ cup of the chopped dates. Process until fine bits form. Place mixture in a bowl along with the juice-water combination.

4. Combine soda, sugar, butter and vanilla in another bowl; mix well.

5. Stir in egg, flour, baking powder and salt. Mix thoroughly. Add nuts.

6. Pour mixture into a 9" x 5" loaf pan; bake for about 50 minutes. Cool 10 minutes. Remove from pan and continue to cool on a rack.

7. Combine confectioners' sugar, grapefruit juice and zest, stirring until it becomes a thin paste. Drizzle over loaf.

Yield: One 9" x 5" loaf.

Grapefruit Marmalade Gingerbread

The enjoyment of this treat is two-fold: First, there's the aromatic gingerbread, and then, the tangy whipped topping. Yum!

1¾ cups cake flour
¾ teaspoon baking powder
½ teaspoon baking soda
1 teaspoon cinnamon
1 teaspoon ground ginger
½ teaspoon salt
3 tablespoons shortening
1 egg, well beaten
½ cup molasses
1 cup grapefruit marmalade
4 tablespoons boiling water
Tangy whipped topping (recipe follows)

1. Preheat oven to 350 degrees F.

2. Spray an 8" × 8" baking pan with non-stick baking spray.

3. Combine baking powder, baking soda, cinnamon, ginger and salt in a large mixing bowl. Set aside.

4. Cream shortening in a large mixing bowl by beating on high until light and fluffy.

5. Add egg; mix well.

6. Add molasses and marmalade; beat thoroughly.

7. Add dry ingredients and hot water alternately in small amounts; beating well after each addition.

8. Pour into the pan; bake for 25 to 30 minutes. Cool for 10 minutes. Cut cake into nine squares and serve with tangy whipped topping.

Servings: 9

Tangy Whipped Topping

What makes this topping so appealing and versatile is that despite its creamy texture, there's a bit of a spike — courtesy of grapefruit.

Whipped Topping:
1 (3-ounce) package cream cheese
1 tablespoon whipping cream
½ teaspoon vanilla extract
3 tablespoons confectioners' sugar

Tangy Grapefruit Sauce:
½ cup sugar
1 tablespoon flour
1 tablespoon cornstarch
⅛ teaspoon salt
¾ cup boiling water
2 tablespoons butter
1 teaspoon grapefruit zest
½ cup grapefruit juice
1 tablespoon lemon juice

1. To create the whipped topping: Bring cream cheese to room temperature. Place in a medium-size mixing bowl along with cream and vanilla extract. Beat until well combined. Gradually blend in the confectioners' sugar; continue to beat until smooth. Set aside.

2. To create tangy grapefruit sauce: Combine sugar, flour, cornstarch and salt in a 2-quart saucepan. Add boiling water and butter. Cook, stirring constantly, over medium heat until thick and clear. Remove from heat. Add zest and fruit juices. Stir to combine. Cool to room temperature.

3. Fold into whipped topping.

Yield: about 2 cups

Grapefruit Mallobet

Mallobets were popular desserts in the late 1940s when home freezer compartments began to expand. Essentially "mallobet" is a composite word "mallo" from marshmallows and "bet" from sherbet. So "mallobet" is essentially sherbet made with marshmallows.

20 marshmallows
1 cup grapefruit juice (divided use)
¼ cup orange juice
2 tablespoons lemon juice
1 tablespoons sugar
½ teaspoon lemon zest
½ teaspoon orange zest
2 egg whites
⅛ teaspoon salt

1. Heat marshmallows and ½ cup grapefruit juice in top of double boiler, folding over and over until marshmallows are half melted.

2. Remove from heat and add remaining grapefruit juice, fruit juices, sugar and zests. Fold over and over until mixture is smooth and spongy. Cool.

3. Beat egg whites until stiff in a medium mixing bowl, and then beat in salt.

4. Fold into fruit mixture.

5. Pour into a refrigerator freezing tray or an 8" × 8" × 2" baking pan. Set in the freezer for about 1½ hours. Stir to keep it from freezing solid. Then freeze for another 1½ to 2 hours.

Servings: 6

Grapefruit Alaska

Grapefruit halves are perfect for individual servings of this show stopping dessert. It's a variation on the classic Baked Alaska, which is a sponge cake layer topped with ice cream and completely blanketed in meringue. Then the confection is baked quickly in a very hot oven until the meringue turns golden before the ice cream melts.

2 chilled pink grapefruit
2 egg whites
2 tablespoons granulated sugar
4 scoops mango sorbet

1. Cut grapefruit in half. Remove center core and free sections from membrane. Refrigerate.

2. Just prior to serving, preheat broiler for 10 minutes.

3. Whip egg whites and granulated sugar into a stiff meringue.

4. Place a scoop of sorbet in center of each of the chilled grapefruit halves.

5. Top each grapefruit half with meringue, taking care to cover the entire top of the grapefruit and seal the edges.

6. Place under a broiler for a minute or two until meringue is lightly browned.

Servings: 6

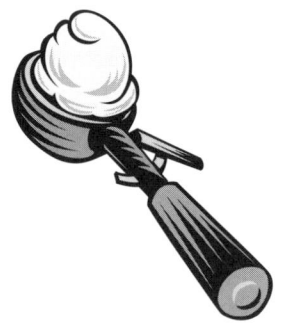

Grapefruit Candy

The secret to success is scraping off all the bitter white pith. It takes a bit of time and trouble, but the results are worth it. In one small mouthful you experience a world of pleasure: The peel is sweet and tender, the hefty grains of turbinado make it crunchy, and the chocolate – well, the chocolate makes it smooth and creamy.

4 grapefruit
Cold water
1½ cups sugar
Rind of ½ lemon
Turbinado sugar (see Note)
Semi-sweet chocolate, melted

1. Peel the grapefruit. Scrape off the white pith. Cut peel into narrow strips.

2. Place in a 2-quart saucepan; cover with cold water and bring to a boil.

3. Pour off the water. Repeat this process three times. Drain well.

4. To make the syrup, combine sugar and 1 cup of water in another saucepan; add juice from grapefruit and the rind of ½ a lemon.

5. Add drained grapefruit zest and boil slowly until all liquid is absorbed, watching the pan carefully to be sure sugar does not burn.

6. Line a cookie sheet with waxed paper or parchment. Dust with turbinado sugar. Place grapefruit strips on the sheet in a single layer, turning to coat well with the sugar. Allow peel to dry overnight.

7. Dip one end of each strip into hot melted semi-sweet chocolate.

Yield: about 2 dozen

Note: Turbinado sugar is a coarse-grained, less refined sugar widely available at supermarkets.

Grapefruit Honey Sticks

*Honey sticks make a great kitchen gift. Excellent for holiday treats;
even young children can help with rolling.*

2 cups orange blossom honey
Juice and zest of one lemon
Juice and zest of one small pink grapefruit
6 teaspoons ground ginger (divided use)
3 to 4 cups matzo meal
½ cup turbinado sugar (see Note)
½ cup chopped pecans

1. Bring honey, fruit juices and zest to a full boil in a 2-quart
saucepan; add 4 teaspoons of the ginger and matzo meal,
stirring until very thick.

2. Combine turbinado sugar with 2 teaspoons of the ginger.
Sprinkle on a baking sheet or waxed paper.

3. Cool honey mixture, then roll between hands into long strips.
Cut into 2-inch pieces.

4. Roll in the sugar-ginger mixture. Store in an airtight container.

Yield: about 2 dozen.

Note: *Turbinado sugar is a less refined sugar widely available in
supermarkets.*

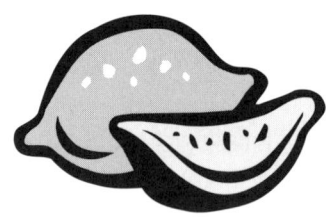

Citrus Nut Sandwich Spread

This is a very tasty sandwich spread that is especially delectable on slices of date or banana bread.

2 (8-ounce) packages cream cheese at room temperature
1 tablespoon grapefruit zest
1 cup cut up orange-scented prunes
½ cup pecans, chopped
½ cup grapefruit juice

1. Cut cream cheese blocks into 8 pieces and place in a food processor bowl.

2. Add remaining ingredients and process until smooth.

Yield: about 2½ cups

Spiced Preserved Grapefruit

You'll be proud to give this as a kitchen gift — especially around the holidays when grapefruit are at their best. Ladled into a pretty jar, and decorated with ribbons, it will please anyone who loves sweet and citrusy things.

¾ cup orange blossom honey
¼ cup lemon juice
1 small grapefruit
¼ cup grapefruit juice
4 whole cloves
1 cinnamon stick

1. Whisk together honey and lemon juice in a 2-quart saucepan until well blended.

2. Cut grapefruit in half lengthwise; cut each half into ¼-inch-thick slices. Stir into honey mix.

3. Add cloves and cinnamon stick; bring mixture a boil over medium heat; reduce heat to low and simmer 10 to 15 minutes or until grapefruit slices are tender. Remove from heat and cool.

4. Place grapefruit and ladle cooking liquid into a decorative container and refrigerate until ready to serve.

Yield: 2¼ cups

Notes

Notes

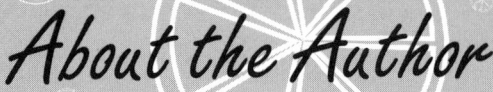

About the Author

Pat Mack, former Food Editor of *The Record* in Hackensack, New Jersey is the recipient of numerous awards from the *Association of Food Journalists*. She has received many citations for her writing as a food journalist and restaurant reviewer, as well as appearing on many television programs, including *The Food Network* and *ABC's Eyewitness News*. Well-known to many professional gastronomes, Pat is also the author of three hardcover cookbooks: *The 15-Minute Chef*, *Tomatoes* (from the kitchen garden to the kitchen table) and *Corn*.

Pat shares her adventures in the culinary while traveling back and forth from her homes in New Jersey and Florida.

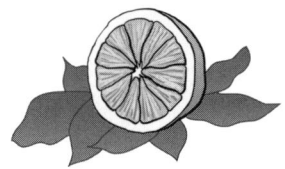